Seeing beyond the Tai Chi Footprint

Sixteen Essential Principles

By

Huan Zhang

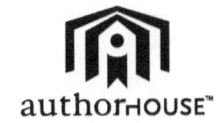

authorHOUSE™

1663 LIBERTY DRIVE, SUITE 200
BLOOMINGTON, INDIANA 47403
(800) 839-8640
WWW.AUTHORHOUSE.COM

First published by AuthorHouse 08/09/05

ISBN: 1-4208-1831-7 (sc)

Printed in the United States of America
Bloomington, Indiana

This book is printed on acid-free paper.

This book is dedicated to my father Lu Ping Zhang, who introduced and taught me his own way of Tai Chi, and my mother Wen Wen Yan, who cooked for me many delicious Chinese meals so that I may have the strength to practice Tai Chi.

Acknowledgment

I would like to thank James Sturnfield for helping to edit this book. He added a lot of good idea and good energy into this book. Without his help, this book won't have been done!

I would also like to thank John Hanson and James, Yael, and Esther Marshall for helping with the some earlier editing of this book.

I would also like to thank William Phillip for writing the comments at the end of this book, Jim Sturnfield who took some of the pictures of my father in this book and shared with me his interpretations of my father's teachings, Bronwen Arthur, Dan Marshall, Jeff Felberbaum and David Grant who volunteered their time to take my pictures.

Table of Contents

I. Preface

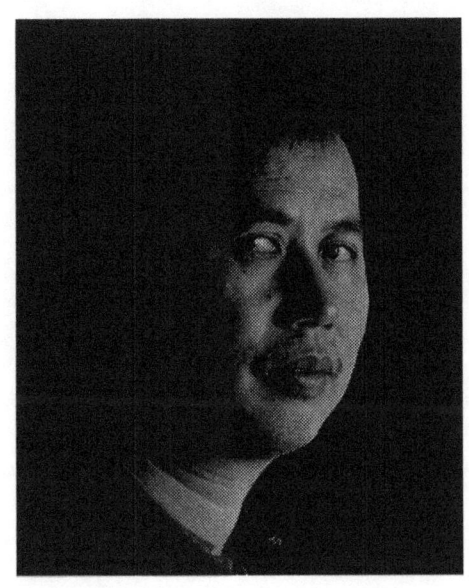

The Request

After my father, Lu Ping Zhang, passed away on April 5, 1998, many of his Tai Chi students asked me if I could record some of my father's Tai Chi theories for them. My father constantly expressed numerous new insights as he taught. He was always helping his students with these theories.

It's almost impossible to put all of his experience, discoveries, and inventions in one book. He knew so many different Chinese martial arts styles such as the five major styles of Tai Chi, various Ba Gua forms, and other Shaolin sets. He studied with many famous and not so famous masters in China who gave him deep insight into the Martial Arts.

Lu Ping's Martial Arts Journey

Lu Ping had begun practicing Martial Arts at an early age. He worked hard and became the head of the Martial Arts club at his school. He used this position to bring in great Martial Artist to teach the club's members. He would find ways to spend private time training and talking with these teachers.

After school, he spent a number of years in the remote countryside. He constantly practiced and searched for other master. His teachers included famous national martial arts champions, the descendents of the founders of many different styles, former policeman, bodyguards and other skilled practitioners.

There is a famous saying in China, "Three people walking, one is my teacher". It means that everywhere there are people with skills to learn. My father told me privately that some teachers who taught him were not good fighters. They did have many other things such as forms or methods that he could utilize to improve his skills. He still paid the respect to these teachers as he would to others who were highly skilled.

Based only on rumors of a great master, he would journey over rough terrain and dangerous wilderness in hope to discover more about the martial arts. His adventures are worthy of a book in themselves.

The Search of "Little Tiger"

One of the examples is his search for a famous master, Chang Hai Seng, whose nickname is "Little Tiger" in the rural state of An Hui. Master Chang Hai Seng was living in the high mountains. In order to find him, my father had to walk many miles. Although he began his trip in the early morning, he could not see any signs of houses as the day turned to evening. The sky was quickly approaching total darkness.

In the dark, he saw some lights and headed towards them. He assumed that these were lights from some houses. He hoped that they might be the lights of master Chang's home. As he approached, the lights moved in different directions. He then could hear the howling of wolves near to him. The lights he had seen were wolves' eyes. He centered himself and stayed on the alert. It was possible that they would attack him if he tried to sleep on the road. He walked quickly away from them and continued on the dark path towards Chang's place.

It was very late when he reached a house. There was only the weak glow of a candle burning. Lu Ping asked if the person he knew where Chang lived. The man asked why he was looking for him and Lu Ping replied that he knew that he was a great martial artist. The man was Chang and expressed his surprise that someone would seek him out because he was in disfavor with the government.

At that time, most people are very poor. China's Cultural Revolution had ruined many people's life and combined with other disasters had left many people with very little for survival. My father had brought Chang a large meal, some provisions and some cigarettes. Master Chang was extremely happy and grateful. Even as he ate this wonderful meal, he started talking with my father and demonstrating with his chopsticks various martial arts movements.

My father was an explorer of the Martial Arts. He was constantly practicing and reading martial arts writings. I can still remember from my early childhood, what an older kid told me about my father. At that time, there were no water faucets in homes. Maybe twenty families would share one outdoor water facet. Every family had a giant stone bowl that would store their water. My father would take water buckets and walk about 15 minutes to the water faucet, fill the buckets and carry them back home. This friend told me, "When I see your father heading to the water faucet, he holds two empty buckets in one hand, and does some kind of strange movements with the other hand. I had thought it was very strange. Finally, I realized he was working on some sort of Martial Arts movement."

Addicted to Martial Arts

One of my father's Tai Chi teachers told me that he had seen my father on the street. My father wasn't paying any attention to his surroundings. He didn't even say hello to his teacher because he was concentrating on a martial art book and reading it while walking. My father was so focused that he appeared unaware that he was headed at a horizontal pole. The teacher was so afraid the Lu Ping would hit it that he shouted a warning to be careful. The teacher concluded that if someone who studied as hard as Lu Ping couldn't figure out a complete martial arts theory, then it couldn't be figured out by anyone. I am sure that even when he was working on his Mathematics, he was thinking about its connection to Martial Arts.

An Honest Teacher

As a believer of Lao Tzu theory, Lu Ping applied his teaching in Lao Tzu's way. In the United States, one of the ways to encourage your students is to please your student. So some teachers will say, "Oh, you are doing good" even though the student did terribly. It's not natural. Lao Tzu's way is to be natural, to be honest and tell the truth. Although some people don't like to have the mistakes in their practice pointed out, the best way to help them improve their Tai Chi is to give honest opinions and to point out their mistakes. Lu Ping did well on this, being natural, being honest, and being really helpful to his student. He used his true heart to help them. He would say, "Oh, you did this terrible, you should do it this way, and practice a hundred times"

He would always be testing his new insights into Tai Chi with his student. He would customize his teaching for each of his student to help them gain their own insights into doing Tai Chi. Often he would show each student a variation of the movements that would aid that student in improving his art. It is thus very challenging to pull these varying concepts together.

Huan's Dream

I dreamed that some day I would produce a book encapsulating my father's principle theories. This book is intended to capture many of the insights into the martial arts that he has expressed. I have taken a number of his major ideas and I have organized them into these sixteen basic principles.

Traditionally, Tai Chi has been transmitted orally and physically. We no longer have the sensational experience neither of doing Tai Chi with my father nor of witnessing the oral lesson being translated into graceful powerful movements. For those who learned from my father, his "song" of Tai Chi, rhythm, music and lyrics are etched in our Psyche. So much is lost when the Master passes away.

This book serves as a partial collection of his knowledge and a reworking of some of his Tai Chi theories. Much of the presentation of these principles is influenced by my own theories and by similar principles that I learned from my other masters. It introduces 16 important principles. It will benefit Tai Chi performers from beginners to advanced-level practitioners, bringing their Tai

Chi to a new level. Each chapter carefully discusses a principle with detailed explanation.

II. Understanding Chinese

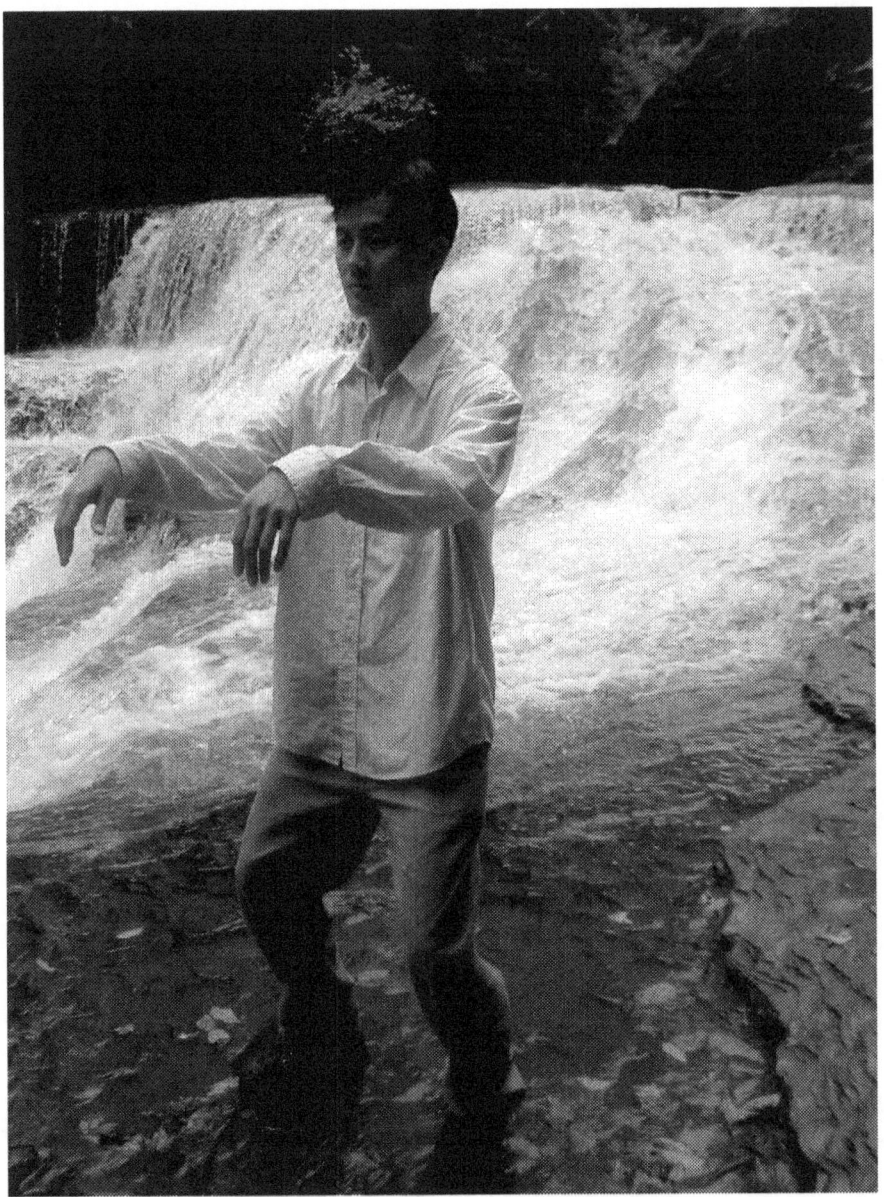

Huan in opening Tai Chi

> "A footprint is formed by a shoe, but how can the footprint be the foot"
>
> Lao Tzu

Trace the Footprint

In the flavor of the above saying, we can consider Tai Chi as the foot and language as the shoe. Chinese and English are different shoes for the foot, so their footprints will be different. This book is from my understanding of Tai Chi and I have expressed my understanding in English. However, Chinese is my mother language and the concepts are Chinese. These concepts formed the roots of an aged tree. They grab tightly in my mind.

In this book, I will try my best to get the natural, original and simplest words to explain Tai Chi without the losing the taste in translating the Chinese to English. I will try to help you see the real foot – Tai Chi.

The Foot and Shoe

It is obvious to say that Chinese is not English, but there are subtleties in the Chinese language that complicate the translation to English or many other languages. The written Chinese language consists of characters that express whole images. Often the use of a particular character expresses not just a word, but also a whole concept with various poetic connections in its thought.

The distinction between male and female pronoun is not placed in the normal Chinese language, so the use of he or she is awkward in a translation. I will often use a masculine pronoun when I would prefer to have a gender-neutral reference. Verbs are not conjugated as in English. I have tried to stay consist in my tense, but I may vary at times between past, present and future.

Another complication occurs because the written language is not phonetic. Some Chinese spoken word could be written with two different characters. It is only the content that determines which one is correct.

The spoken language has been given various transliterations into English sound. These phonetic transformations have problems because they often mislead an English speaker into completely mispronouncing a word and usually lack the tonal information that would distinguish it from a similar word. Two different words can have the same sounds except for tonal quality, so an English transliteration does not naturally carry this information and care must be used in their interpretation.

I will use different transliterate words for the same because of the varied ways which I have seen them expressed in English. For example, "Chi" and "Qi" are actually different transliterates of the same Chinese word. I will use these as they have often been used; Qi will be used when I use the Chinese expression for energy while Chi will be used in the concept of Tai Chi. (The chi in "Tai Chi" and Qi in qi kung, are different letters in Chinese).

III. Tai Chi and Energy

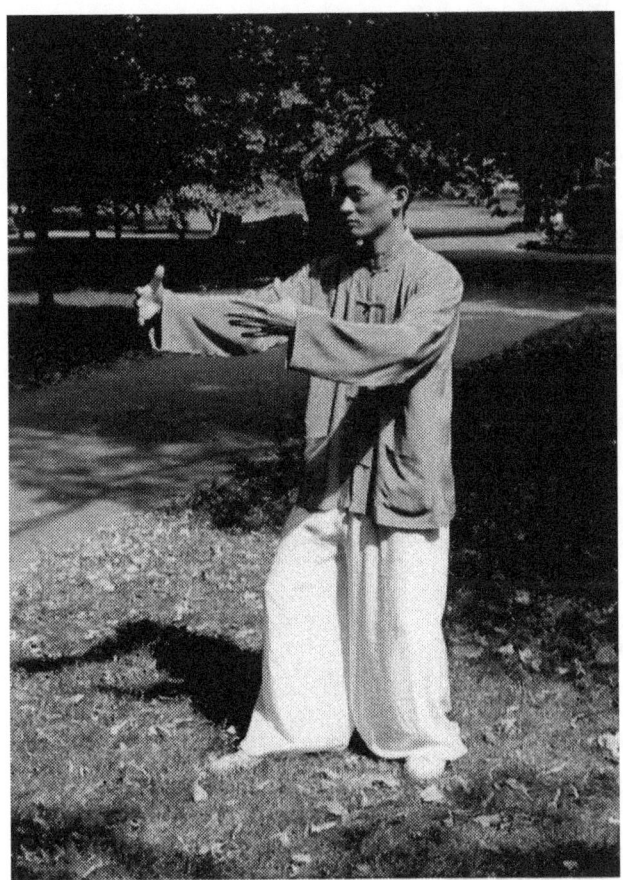

Huan in energy training gesture

"For a human who often moves, the bad energy will be gone, the blood will circulate properly. He will not get sick, his body will not quickly approach the end of its lifetime"

Hua Tuo as translated by Huan Zhang.

Hua Tuo's Wisdom

One thousand and five hundred years ago (Han Dynasty), the greatest doctor in Chinese history, "Magic Doctor" Hua Tuo made the above statement about moving exercises. Hua Tuo's statement has been proved with many exercises, especially with Tai Chi. This statement tells us that when humans do exercises, the bad Qi (energy) will be gone and the good Qi will be created. This improves the health of the person.

Tai Chi is not only an ancient Chinese exercise. It is also a martial arts form that involves a relaxed whole body rotation, the concentration of the mind, and body balance. The commonly known benefits of Tai Chi are relaxation and better overall health. Some people also discover the self-defense aspects of its practice and the confidence that it provides.

Typical Tai Chi, Energy, and Health Questions

In order to expand on the relationship between Tai Chi and energy, we will look at some typical questions about Tai Chi, energy, and health.

Is there any proof that Tai Chi really improves one's health?

There are many stories about how practicing Tai Chi has helped various people overcome health problems. I have seen many people become healthy and stronger from doing Tai Chi regularly. I have even known of people who health seemed to improve from regularly watching someone do Tai Chi. There have been scientific studies showing that Tai Chi improves kinetic balance and reduces the occurrence of falls.

Will Tai Chi practice improve everyone's health?

The improved energy flow from doing Tai Chi is beneficial for everybody. It is never certain if the damage that the body has sustained over it years or from genetic weakness can be over come by this improved energy. I believe that doing Tai Chi does extend life and improve health. In some cases, it may not overcome the existing problems, but I imagine that things would have been worst if Tai Chi hadn't been practiced.

How does Tai Chi increase your health?

A Tai Chi practice cause the body to takes in, store, and increases its energy. It improves the alignment and integration of the body. It allows the body to relax so that the internal organs can be healthier.

How do people get their energy?

People get their energy from many different ways. Basically, it can be divided into four different categories: by breathing, relaxing, feeding yourself, and doing exercise. Tai Chi is related to all these four categories.

Tai Chi coordinates the breath with the body movements to allow deeper and richer intake of air. It allows better alignment, so that the blood circulation system, lymphatic system, nervous system and the meridian system (Chi flow) can flow freely.

Tai Chi relaxes the mind and body. This allows the muscles to remove toxin and increase their energy and allows the mind to revive itself as in rest. The relaxation also allows the organs to get more blood and process food more effectively.

Performing Tai Chi involves doing a coordinated exercise that involves the whole body. It tones and develops the whole body.

How does your body recharge its energy?

Usually, your body recharges its energy while you sleep or take a rest. Good sleep requires good breathing, relaxing, and some food in the stomach. If you can't breathe well, you will not be able to sleep well. If you cannot get relaxed, it will also affect your sleep.

There most certainly have been times when you can't sleep well. You may have slept on the floor one or more times in your life and found that you couldn't relax because your back felt stiff against the hard floor. You may have gone to bed feeling hungry or thirsty and found that you couldn't settle down. You feel tired after a bad night's sleep; on the other hand, if you have been properly nourished and have gotten a good night sleep you will awake full of energy because you have recharged your body energy properly.

In the same way as sleep, Tai Chi involves good breath and relaxation of body. It is an exercise that does the same thing for you as sleep or taking a rest. We can also say Tai Chi is a way of resting your body and mind. Resting or relaxing is like recharging a battery. When you do Tai Chi, your body transfers the elements and nutrition you have received from food to energy. That's why we say, feeding yourself is also related to Tai Chi because, without eating, you have no strength to do Tai Chi and, without Tai Chi, you miss a good way to transfer your food to good energy.

What's the difference between being young and being old?

Gray hair comes out when a person is getting old. It shows that your body doesn't have enough energy to reproduce parts of your body perfectly such as dark hair. The older person is not as energetic as before.

A leaf on a branch is fresh and soft. As it gets older, it loosens its grip on the limb. A wind can pull it from the tree. Without the sap from the tree, it turns yellow and crisp; it loses its energy and dies.

For a person, it's the same thing. When a person is young, he has a lot of energy, his skin and body is soft; on the other hand, the skin becomes drier, hard, and wrinkled with age. Tai Chi practice makes the body more energetic and reverses the aging process. It can soften the body and delay the hardness and stiffness associated with getting older.

Can you hurt yourself if you do Tai Chi wrong?

Certainly, Tai Chi is good for most people. But if not done properly or if not modified properly for a person's current condition, it could lead to problems. Because it is done gently, it is less likely to cause problems than other exercises. Special care and awareness should be given to the alignment of the knees since this is the one place where injuries have occurred.

How does one know if Tai Chi is being done correctly?

Understanding and applying the principles of Tai Chi will help to insure that it is being done correctly. One should pay attention to how the body feels and seek out experience teachers to help guide the correct practice.

Now that you probably have a better idea of how Tai Chi can help you, I will introduce to you some important principles about Tai Chi to help and improve your Tai Chi performance. These principles include how to use your eyes, feet, fingers, hands and arms in Tai Chi performance. They also teach you how to relax and to control your weight and timing. The principles even involve advanced theories that will constantly challenge the practitioner to new levels of skill.

IV. The Principles

1. Relaxing the Right Way

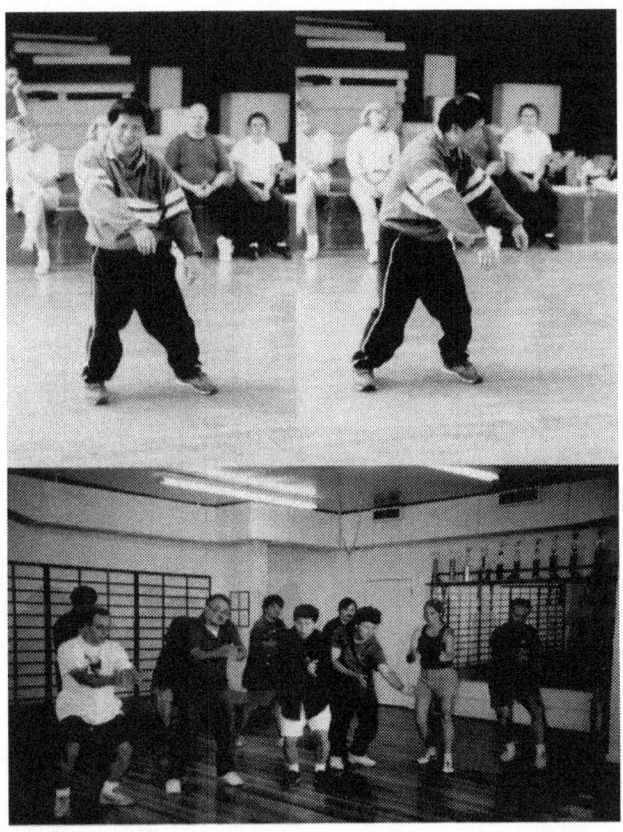

Master Lu Ping Zhang shows students a special exercise to relax their spine.

> "Increasing the ability to relax the joints should be a natural progression and thus stretching and extension should not be overdone."
>
> Zhang, Lu Ping[1]

Many people get involved in Tai Chi because they are very stressed, with a lot of pressure from work or school. They want to learn the right way to relax. They want to learn some magic way to be healthy.

It is easy to say the word "relax," but, when you really try to do it, it's very hard to even realize that you are not relaxed. Most people think they can relax, but they only relax part of their body. Usually one part of the body is partly relaxed while other parts are still stressed. For example, your arms are relaxed, but your shoulders might be tight. Your shoulders are relaxed, but your back might be stressful.

When most people relax, they fall into their underlying state of tension. The tightest muscles do not release at all and other muscles can't fully release because they need to maintain a balance in the body structure. Still other muscles are tightening to allow some muscles to let go.

To truly relax, the body has to have the right shape, alignment, and connection. Shorten muscles are not relaxed. They will lengthen and stretch as they relax. The joints will be free and loose because they are not compressed by contracting muscles. The body will only engage the minimum needs to maintain its shape.

At the beginning stage, your body is not ready to relax and open fully for you; you need to use Tai Chi to help you to relax your whole body.

Basically, relaxation can be reached by two different ways, one is body stretch and another is mind concentration. Meditation forms such as yoga do a lot of stretch work in order to relax. What is stretching? It's a way to soften your veins and spine. It is a way to extend your muscles and joints. It's a way to open your body. It's a way to get you relaxed for the next stage.

If you see an old person, when he walks on the street, his back is humble and his head is looking down. His arms are pulled tight to his body. That's the opposite of stretch. Once you are well stretched, then your arms and legs can be looser. When you are relaxed, your arms are stretched and can reach further.

The Rats and Tiger in Your Mind

Now, let's talk about how mind concentration helps you relax. Using your mind to control the level of relaxation in your body is a traditional way of Qi Kung, which is a breathing and relaxation exercise. It is best to get rid of messy thinking and to try to empty your mind and be at peace with yourself.

I will tell a very famous Chinese Buddhist story that reflects on the power of the mind. A hiker was walking along a mountain. Suddenly, he slipped and slid off the edge of the Mountain. He had much tension while he was sliding, but his hand was relaxed enough to be open. Fortunately, he was therefore able to grab a long vine when he slipped to it. After he knew he was safe, he felt more relaxed. Suddenly, he heard growls down under his feet. He realized there was a tiger under his feet down the mountain looking at him, so he again felt tense. He was afraid of being eaten by the tiger if he didn't keep a tight grip on the vine. After he climbed up a little more and saw the tiger become smaller under his eyes, he felt relaxed again.

Unfortunately, he found that two rats were gnawing at the vine on the edge of the mountain, so he was frightened again that the vine rope would break and he would fall into the mouth of the tiger. Meanwhile, he smelled a very good, fresh scent. He looked straight ahead and saw two wild strawberries growing out of the stones from the wall of the mountain. He stretched one of his arms, slowly picked them, and put them into his mouth. They tasted so delicious. With this experience, he realized the meaning of his whole life and he became totally relaxed.

This example tells you that your mind controls the way you feel your body. Now, we know that tension is just a way your mind acts. If your mind can relax, then your body will relax as well. As the Buddhist holy books said, the evil is from your heart and mind. To empty the evil, you have to empty your mind and heart. The things you see with your eyes, the sounds you hear with your ears, the odors you smell with your nose, they all come to your mind and create a fake vision to disturb your relaxation and make you feel tension. I want to say that, in order to get rid of your tension; you must empty your mind.

The Procedures of Body Relaxation

If you want to achieve whole body relaxation, you need to empty your mind first. After your mind quiets down, try to relax the top of your head and your forehead. Next, let your mind relax the muscles of your face and then your neck. Continue your mind focus down your body. After you have relaxed your shoulders and your spine, let the relaxation spread out the whole arm, through the wrist, through the whole hand, and out the fingers. Feel the fullness of the relaxation in the upper body and then let it move down the legs, through the knees, through the foot and out the toes.

An important reminder is that relaxation in Tai Chi doesn't mean to let your body fall like mud or melt like ice cream. These are not feelings of complete relaxation. The body has a natural structure so it must be in proper balance.

If an individual muscle loses all its tone, other muscles become tense and stiff to hold the body in balance. If a group of surface muscles are overly loose, then deeper muscles may be overly tight to hold the body structure. As all the muscle relax in unison, the muscles are longer and the joints can open up.

With repeated practice of Tai Chi, the body will begin to relax. By using the mind, the relaxation will become deeper. By keeping the correct shape, the tighter muscles will be stretched. The slow movements of Tai Chi allow the mind to guide the body so that it maintains the correct shape, which in turn will stretch the different parts of the body.

The Lazy Person

Another view that the mind can use to deepen relaxation is to imagine oneself as an extremely lazy person. Each movement of the form is being done with as little additional effort as is possible. The act of lifting an arm or leg should feel as if is almost impossible. No unnecessary muscles should be trying to help the effort of raising the limb.

Even the act of standing should feel as if it is almost impossible. The lower back should not tighten up to support weight. The legs should solely support the body. The thighs and hamstrings should feel warm with the demand of their use.

With this practice, the maximum amount of the body will be relaxed. All the joints should be free to move. The maximum amount of the body will be free to respond to any changes.

2. Using Breathe Control

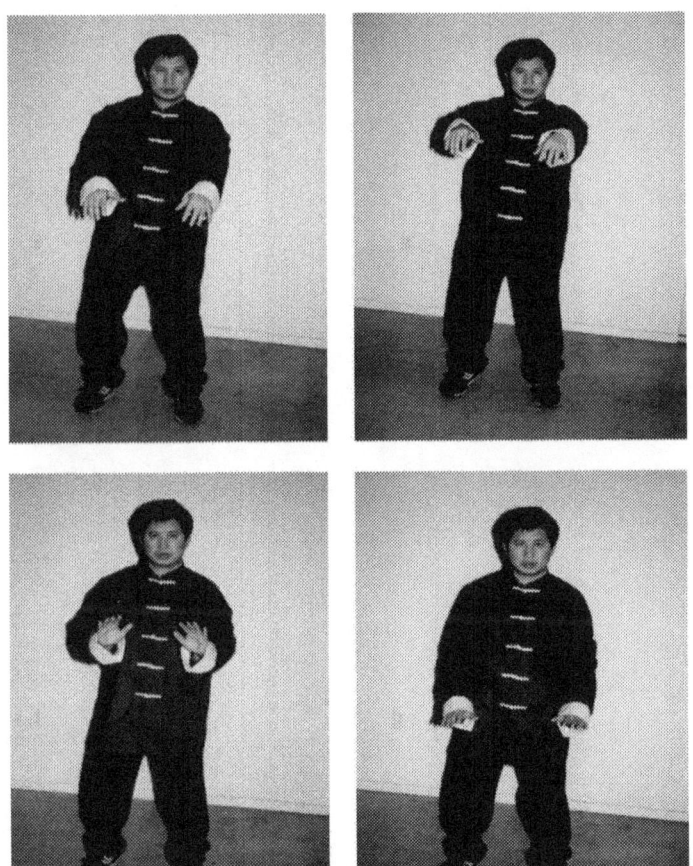

Master Lu Ping performs apply breathing exercise in opening form.

"To open up your body to the chi energy, you must breathe, as we say, like an unborn baby. It's no use forcing anything, like your breathing or movements, as you will only encounter resistance. Instead, you must induce."

Lu Ping Zhang[2]

Control Your Breath

A very important thing is to have good breath control such as the breathing you would do in Yoga and some other meditation styles. You can develop good breathing through practicing Tai Chi. To follow the slow movement, you need to breathe long and slowly to follow the gestures and steps.

It is also important not to fight or hold your breath. The breath should become slower not because you want to match the slow movement, but because it has become deeper and more relaxed. If the breath does not yet match the movements, do not force the breathing. Allow yourself to breathe extra times with a movement. It is more important to have a regular, good breath then it is to synchronize it with the movements.

Many people wonder when you need to breathe in and when you need to breathe out. The best answer for that is Tai Chi has many movements: each movement can be considered as alternating between opening and closing. You are open and tend to breathe out when in gestures such as the standing gestures of "White Crane spreads its Wings" when the hand moves up or "Single Whip" as the arms move apart. On the other hand, you tend to breathe in when you have a closed gesture such as "Lifting Hands" while the one hand moves towards the elbow and "Fist under Elbow" while the fist moves towards the elbow.

"Human's life is between your breaths." Buddha, the creator of Buddhism

One day, Buddha asked his students, "How long is a human's life?"

"50 years?"

"No."

"40 years?"

"No."

"Well, how long is a human's life?"

"It's between your breaths," He answered.

Breathe In and Breathe Out

What is the difference between breathing in and breathing out? Breathing in should bring to mind the ideas of "up, raise, yield, and store." When you breathe in, your muscles tend up and your chest has the feeling of rising, your body has the feeling of yielding to the breath, and you store the Qi. Breathing out should bring to mind the ideas of "down, fall, strength, and release." When you breathe out, your muscles tend to go down, your chest tends to fall, your body feels strengthened, and you are releasing your Qi.

The breath has to be "slow, even, deep, thin, and long." "Slow" obviously means you breathe slowly. "Even" means every breath has to be equal. "Deep" means you have to completely breathe in and out - don't breathe half in and half out. "Thin" means your mouth shouldn't be wide open when you breathe. "Long" means you need to use long breathing instead of short breathing.

Because of body conditions and other activities, some people learn to breathe very long, such as swimmers and divers; others breathe very short and fast, such as runners and basketball players. Some people want to apply one way of breathing in one movement and another way of breathing out in another movement, so sometimes if the movement is too long they tend to hold their breath until they finish certain movements, and this is a big mistake. Holding your breath will cause tension of the muscles and chest. It will change your concentration and relaxation.

Another mistake is breathing too heavily. That's another difference between Tai Chi and other external sports such as tennis, basketball, and soccer. Instead of the breath being heavy, rapid, and strong, the breath has to be quiet, easy, and relaxed. Only by breathing easily, relaxed, and slowly, will the breathing not hurt the body's internal organs. As Lu Ping said, you need to learn how to breathe like an unborn baby.

> "Don't think about the Chi and don't think about the breath. Just perform. Just make yourself relaxed without laws. That's the best law."
>
> Zhang, Lu Ping[3]

Breathe Naturally

Another common way to develop the breath is to breathe naturally without worrying about following the movements. That's the way my father really suggests. "Breathe like an unborn baby" or "don't think about breath" really means to breathe naturally. Some people emphasize too much on breathing, which takes attention away from concentrating on relaxing and the right movement. That's a big mistake many people make.

Returning to the question of when to breathe in and when to breathe out, one should be aware that there are actually three different philosophies that are correct. The previous paragraph shows one of these. The breath is independent of the movement. This philosophy allows the breath to develop naturally and keeps ones from interfering with their own energy. It also keeps an opponent from predicting the timing of a movement from the rhythm of the breath.

Another method, which hasn't been mention, uses the breath to aid the movement in the opposite way from the best method first given. With this approach, the inhale accompanies the raising of the hand so the lifting of the chest in the inhale extends to the lifting of the arm. When closing such as in "Press", this approach would exhale so that the collapsing of the chest would match the compression in the body. This may at first be a more natural action, but an opponent can take advantage of these extremes. The best approach keeps a balance of the breath with the body motion so that the opponent cannot take advantage of extremes.

Good breath can help you in life. There are many systems that focus on the importance of breath. As an example: a very Famous Shao Lin breathing exercise from Shao Lin temple in China is Yi Jin Jing (the bible of "Changing Vine"). It strictly concentrates on breathing. These exercises help develop stronger muscles and healthier inside organs. Good breathing can massage your stomach and chest. It can also bring the Qi to Dan Tian, a spot below the belly where you store your energy and Qi. Good breath can release your stress.

Another thing you should pay attention to is where and when you do Tai Chi. You want to perform it in some place with fresh and good air, such as in a park with trees around or near the water with fresh air. When you breathe, you breathe in good oxygen and breathe out the body's waste products. The best time for doing breathing in Tai Chi is usually in the air of early morning and late night that is fresh and clean.

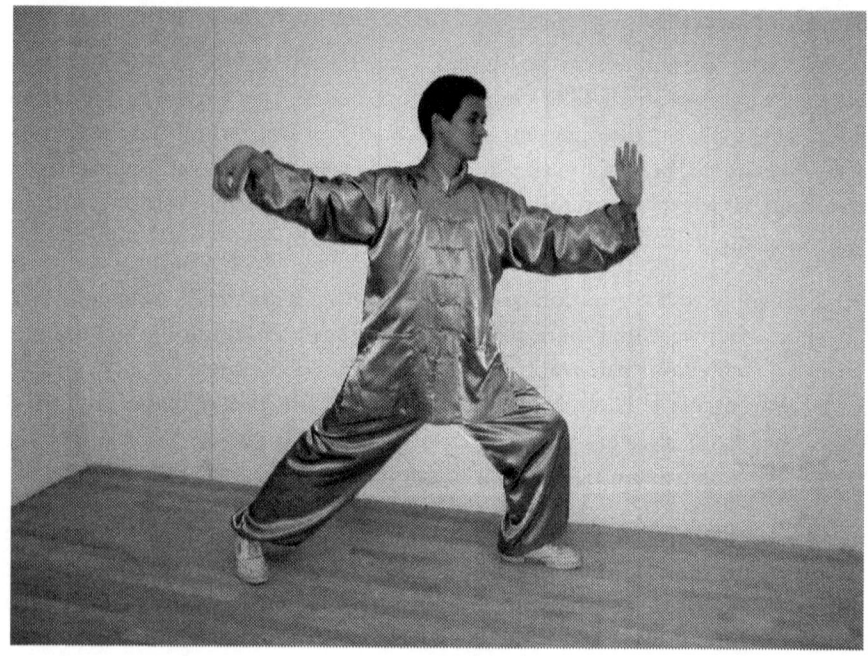

Single Whip

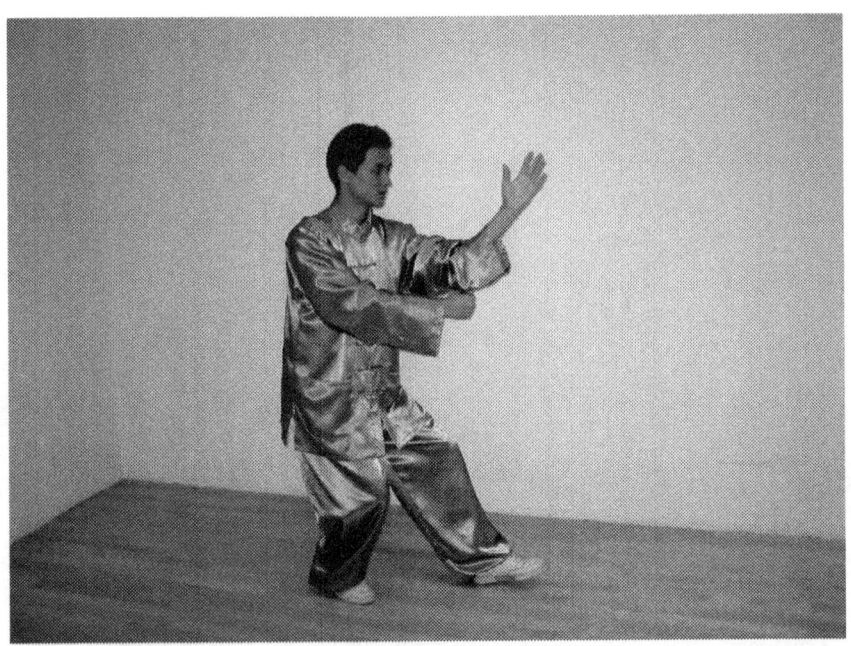

Fist Under Elbow

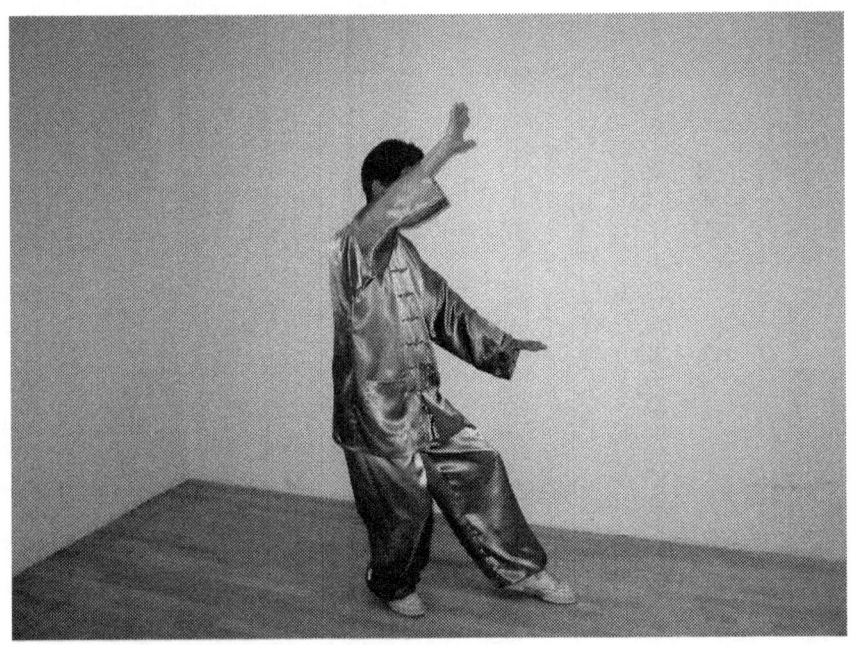

White Crane Spread It's Wings

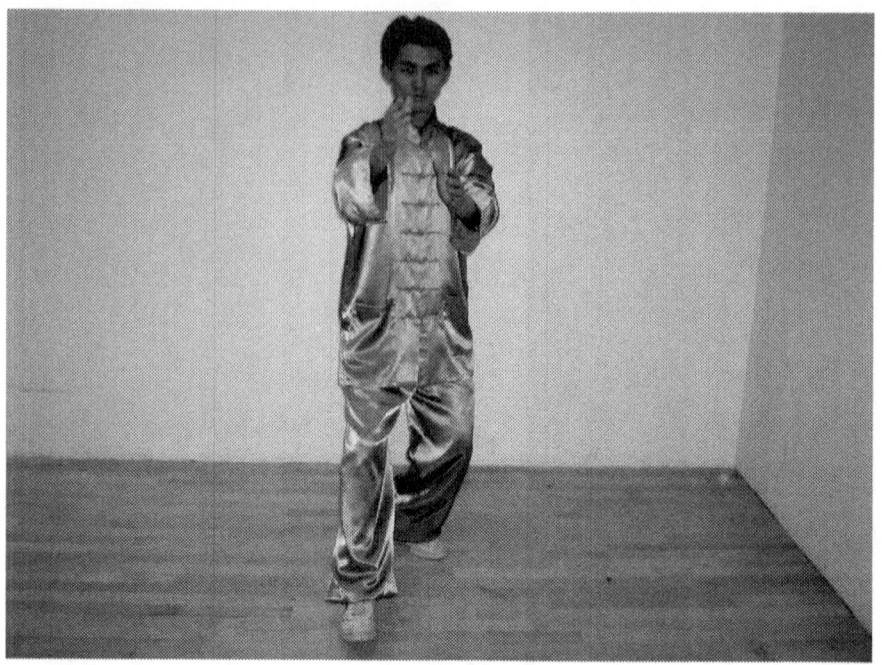

Lifting Hands

3. *Making Scrambled Eggs*

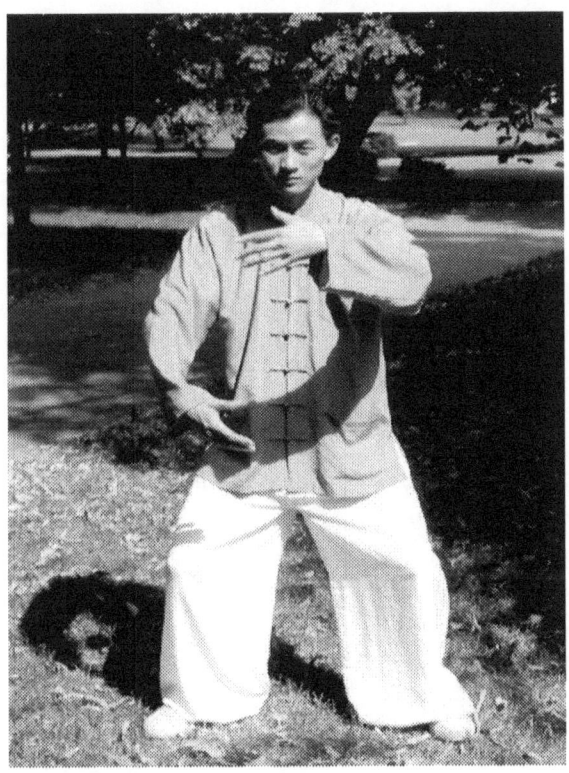

Huan Zhang practice waving hands like moving clouds.

> "The sky and earth are huge, but their activities and changes are balanced and even"
>
> Chuang Tzu

Smooth Your Scrambled Eggs

The speed of Tai Chi is like scrambled eggs. You need to evenly spread the salt on them, so you will get the perfect taste. Abruptness does not really help with cooking the eggs evenly. It requires certain smoothness regardless of being done either slow or fast.

To get the most out of your Tai Chi practice, you have to perform your movements evenly. There is a need to be diligent in ones performance and keep the speed constant. Often a practitioner will move slowly in the places where they are focused, but will speed up as they move their attention to the movement beyond what they are doing.

For examples, consider movements that are repeated like "brush knees" and "waving hands like moving clouds". Each of these repetitions should be performed at the same speed. As the last repetition is started, it is easy to start thinking about the next movement. The current movement doesn't have the same attention as the other repetitions did and will tend to be done more quickly.

You also have to pay attention to the speed between different sets of movements. A lot of people practice slowly on some more mediated movements such as "repulse monkey", "waving hands like moving clouds", but they go faster on more application oriented movement such as "grasp the bird tail" or "single whip". Of course, the distinction between mediated and applied is a false perception and each movement should be treated with the same respect and evenness.

Just imagine if you cooked scrambled eggs and you didn't spread the salt out evenly; some part would have no taste and some part would be too salty. That would be a bad experience for you and others who tried to enjoy your cooking. You don't want your Tai Chi to taste like "bad" scrambled eggs. Only when you pay attention to every individual movement and try to do it evenly, will you start practicing the whole Tai Chi set well.

Time Control

"As a beginner, you may perform Tai Chi for as little as 15 minutes. However, as you progress you will perform for 20 minutes. Eventually, you will perform as long as 40 minutes."

Zhang Lu Ping[4]

If you didn't spend enough time frying your scrambled eggs, they might be raw and you might get diarrhea from them. You need to spend more time to cook them well. You need to cook them on the right heat and scrambled them properly to insured that they are right.

A lot of students have asked questions such as "how long should you spend to finish one set of Tai Chi?" or "How fast or slow should you do it?" Many masters will give you different answers since so many factors are involved. It depends on the many different ways people perform and what level they are at.

If you really need a certain answer, then I would have to say it usually depends on how long the Tai Chi set is. Of course, you will take less time for short forms such as the simplified Tai Chi form and you will take more time for long forms such as Chen Style Tai Chi. A good time frame is 20 minutes for sets such as the 85 movement set of Yang Style Tai Chi. If you do it too fast, you probably don't have enough time to concentrate on each individual movement.

Also your body won't get enough practice if you are too fast. This is not a matter of the total time that you practice. It is much more of a work out to do a simplified form once in fifteen minutes than to do it twice in the same time frame. To do it slow, forces every part of the body to be involved with the movement while going fast allows some parts of the body to coast through on the work of other muscles.

Fast is easy and slow is difficult. Just as when you drive a car, you need patience if traffic moves slowly. It can require more concentration and acceptance of the time needed to complete your journey.

I encourage students to keep trying to do it a little slower, so they will get a real practice on each movement. It becomes a way of meditation that trains your patience. Only by becoming very patient will you then be able to perform the movements well. Without patience and detail, Tai Chi can't be done beautifully.

If you are not patient and eat your burger very fast, you might find that you did not digest it very well. Tai Chi is the same thing; it takes time to make it perfect.

Should you immediately start taking an hour to do the form? Well, let's assume you are regularly running. If you decide to run 10 miles instead of 1 mile a day, you will notice the challenge. You may be able to run it, but you may also injure you body. Will your body maintain the proper stride? How best to increase the endurance will depend on the individual.

How much time do you think you will have to practice Tai Chi everyday? Don't be greedy. Start with appropriate time that you know that you will give to it regularly and then build up.

Also, it is a mistake to do Tai Chi extremely slow because you are supposed to do it slowly. It will not be Tai Chi any more. If you perform for more than one hour, the movement may be stagnating. It will become something like meditating in a Qi Kung form, which emphasizes slow or still movements.

Finally, you can always try different speeds to find the best time for yourself. Each different speed will show you different challenges.

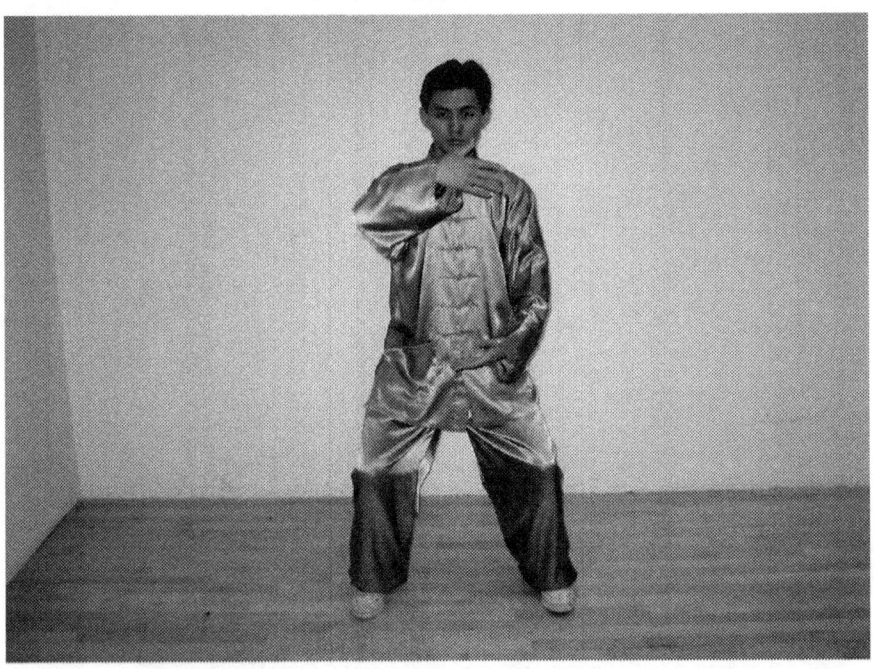

Wave Hands Like Moving Clouds

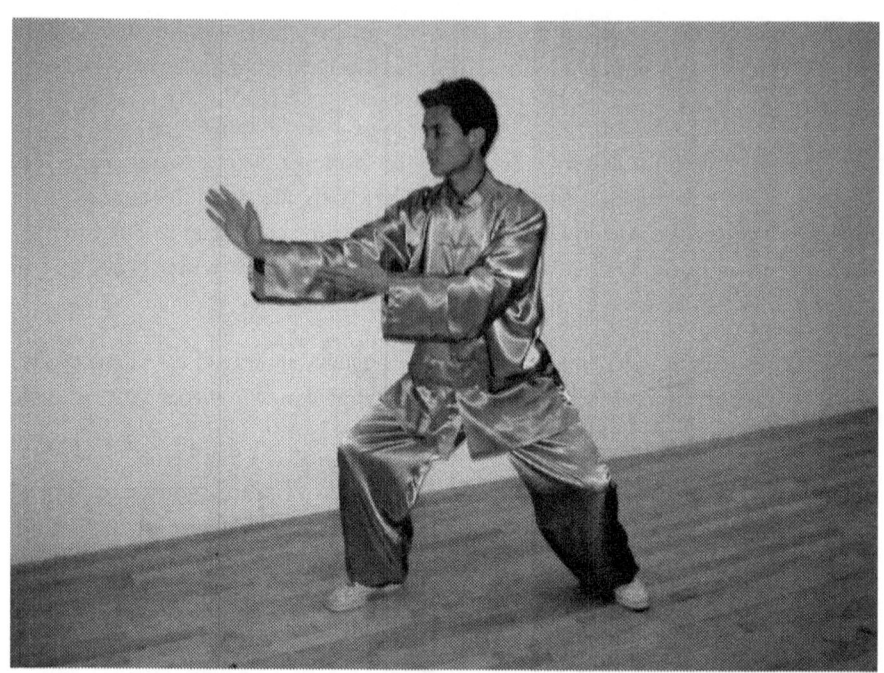

Brush Peacock's Tail - Lu

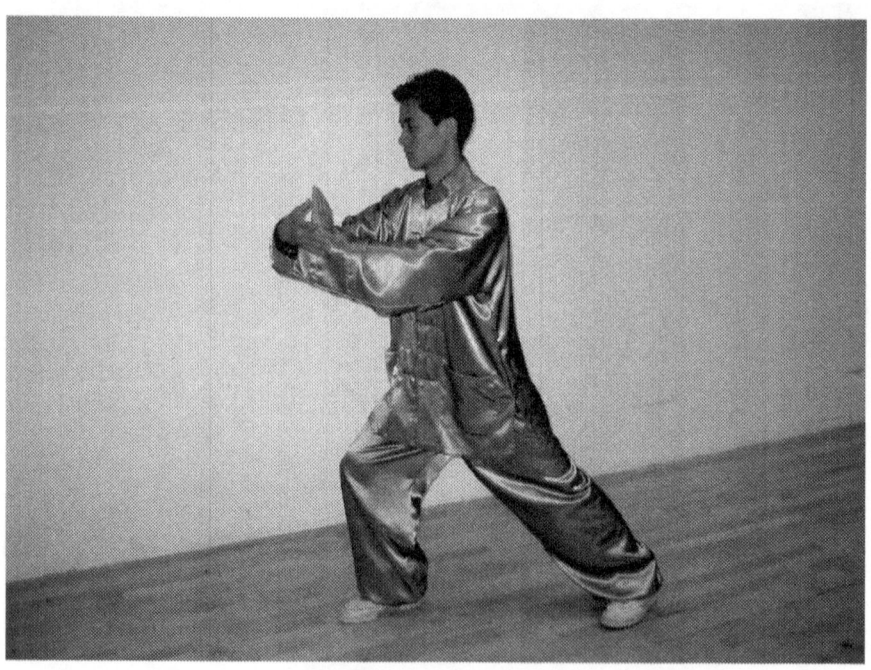

Brush Peacock's Tail - Ji

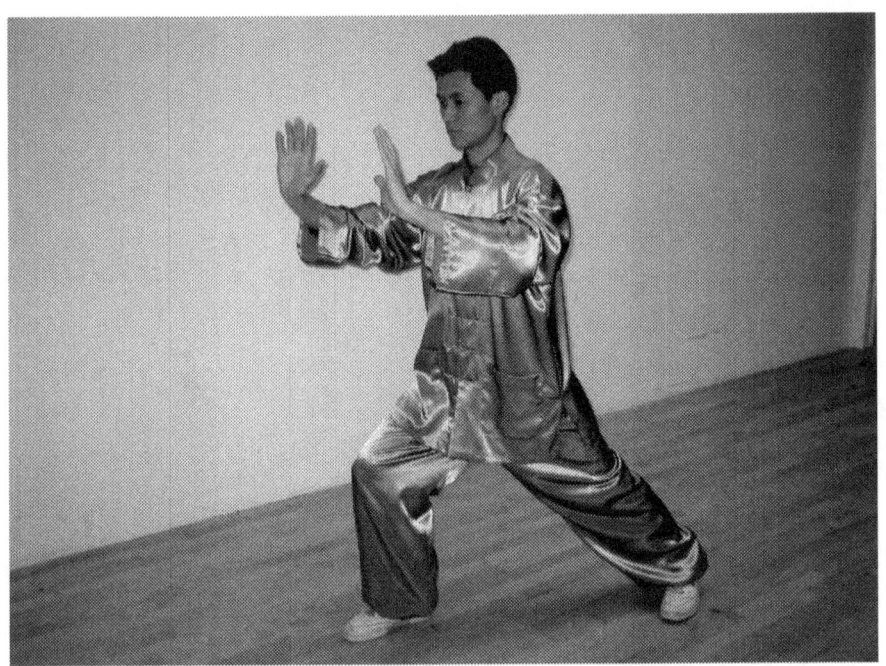

Brush Peacock's Tail - An

4. Making Chinese Noodle

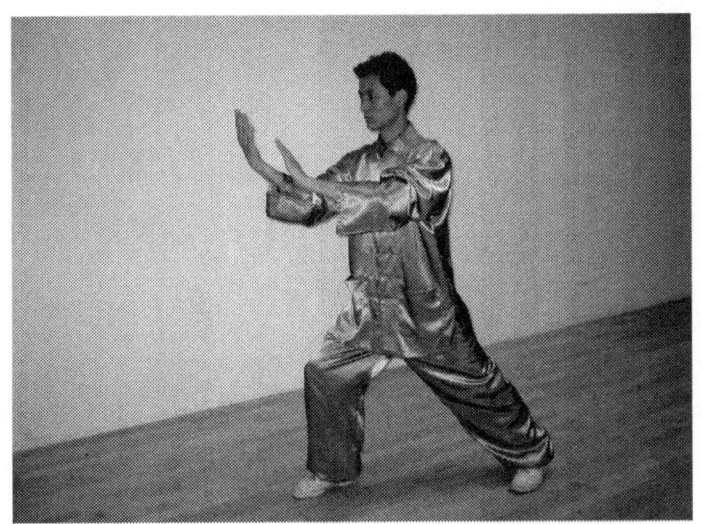

Huan Zhang uses noodle theory in Peng

> "Cai Feng Xiang is the greatest living champion in China. His Legs look like noodles when he kicks."
>
> Lu Ping Zhang[5]

Grandmaster Cai used to tell me that the legs in martial arts must be like Chinese Noodles. Because he practiced "baby's leg" since he was a child, his legs were very flexible. He used to have a nickname, "the fast leg." Five years ago when I met him again, he was 68; he still had such fast reactions and was able to wrap his legs around your shoulders and arms.

At a seminar, he asked someone to punch at him. He kicked up his leg and wrapped it around the arm, catching the punch and holding on to his attacker. He continued to talk with the other students as he held the arm with his leg. When he finished talking, he shook his leg and sent the puncher flying back. The puncher later commented that he wasn't able to pull his arm away from the leg.

My father also used this theory but emphasized the arms should also be like Chinese noodles. Let me use Chinese noodles and uncooked spaghetti as an example to show you the difference between the arms we want to have and the arms we want to develop.

What's the difference between Chinese noodles and uncooked spaghetti? When the noodle and spaghetti are cold, you can't stretch spaghetti but you can stretch the Chinese noodle. What if you bend the spaghetti? It will break, but the Chinese noodle will not because it is soft while the spaghetti is hard.

When you eat Chinese noodles, they drape down from the chopsticks. If you use a fork, you can twirl them around. As you lift them from the plate, you sometimes have to pull at it to separate it from the rest of the noodles. This showed that Chinese noodles have the flexibility to stretch. If you press on a pile of noodle, it will spring back when you release. This shows that they also contain bouncing ability.

Apply this theory to Tai Chi. Your arms need to be soft and flexible like the Chinese noodle when you are making moves. It will contain both the softness and toughness. It can bounce forward and backward.

Now you know the real "taste" of the Chinese noodle. When you go to a Chinese restaurant next time, order some Chinese noodles to eat; you might get a better understanding of a new Tai Chi theory.

While practicing hand exercises like Peng, Lu, Ji and An, you can really apply the "Chinese noodle" theory. In order to make your arms like a Chinese noodle, you need to concentrate, relax, and loosen your muscles, stretch your arms, and imagine your hands and arms like these magical Chinese noodles. Good and constant practice of this theory will soften your hands and arms and flex your arms and body.

5. *Walking at the Edge on the Top of the Empire State Building*

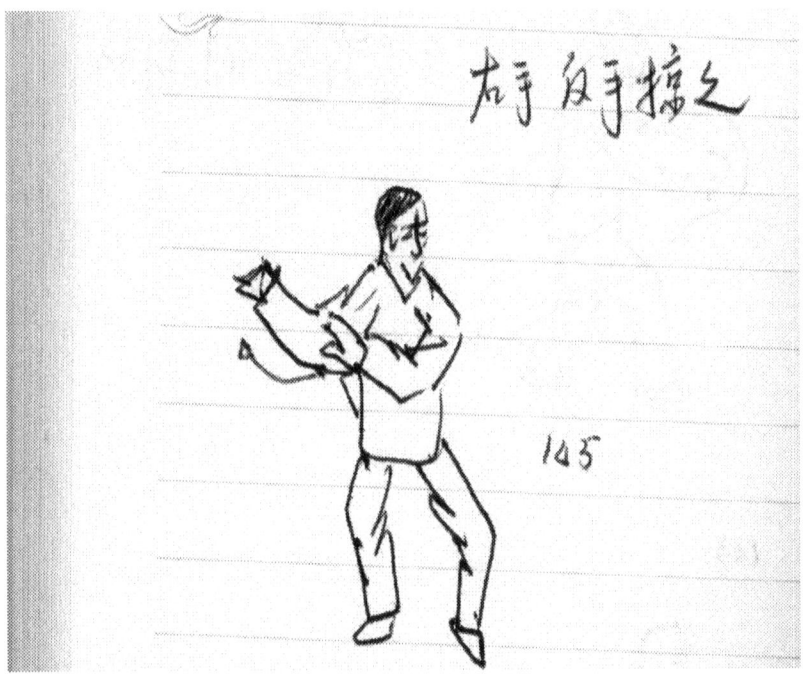

A Snapshot from Master Lu Ping Zhang's drawing/notebook of how carefully you should put down your feet on brush knee.

"Sickness will visit you when you are older, because you didn't take care of your body when you were young. The troubles you have which bring you down, are the troubles you got when you were growing. As a human being in your life, you need to feel like you are holding a glass full of liquid. You need walk extremely carefully, so it won't leak."

Hong Ying Min[6]

Doing Tai Chi is the same as staying a good healthy human being. You need extra care and sense. The foundation for the body is the feet. If you are going to take care with how you move through life, you have to make sure that you take care with how you place your feet.

How are you going to walk if you walk on the edge of the top of the Empire State Building? You might say, be aware, or be careful, or step accurately, so you don't fall. Yes, the position of your feet is very important in Tai Chi. Random steps can destroy the whole Tai Chi practice. The step controls the movement of Tai Chi. It controls the force and direction of Tai Chi and, since it's part of your body, it will affect your arm and body movements. Accuracy is the key for Tai Chi steps.

In some movements, one foot supports the body's weight while the other foot potentially supports the hand against an opponent or the body against the wind. Both feet should not be on the same line in gestures like "brush knee" or "obliquely flying"(Draw 5-1). The feet need to be space far enough apart and angled in a way to allow the hips to be open and for the tailbone to hang freely. If both feet are on the same line, it's not strong enough to support your body against the "winds". To check your feet position, when you move your front foot to line up with your back foot, they should have at least one fist distance.

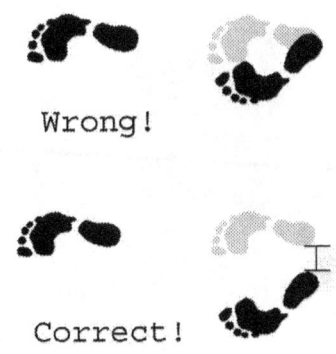

Wrong!

Correct!

In some movements, your feet need to be parallel in order to maintain the Qi. For example, in the opening form, both feet have to be parallel with shoulder width in order to have a good stance to relax and to have good Qi. Another example is the "repulse monkey" gesture in which you turn the heel of your front foot to keep parallel with the back foot in order to maintain balance and move the Qi to your hands.

In some movements, you need to concentrate more weight on one leg than the other; for example, in "pat the high horse", "raise hands", "step to seven stars" and "playing the Pipa". To maintain accurate movements, you need to know which leg to put more weight on and which leg to put less weight on. A common mistake is to have your weight equally distributed.

One foot carries all the weight in other movements, such as "right heel kick, left turn on right heel and left heel kick", "Golden cock stands on right and left leg", and "sweep the lotus leg". In order to do such movements well, your balance must be accurate and even. The force and weight on your legs must be well placed; don't lean forwards or backwards.

Remember you are on the edge of the Empire State Building and you don't want to take a risk in falling off.

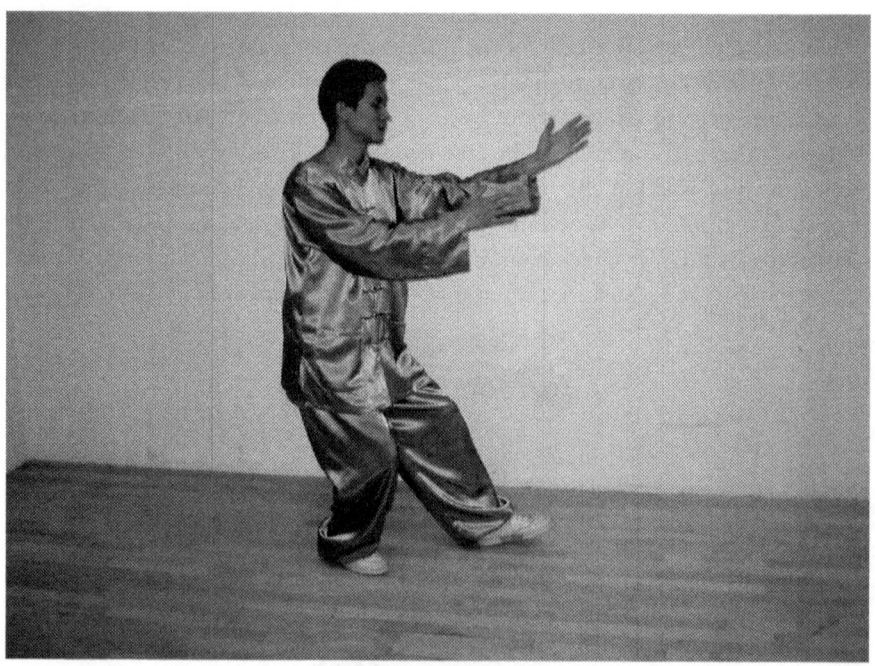

Playing Pipa

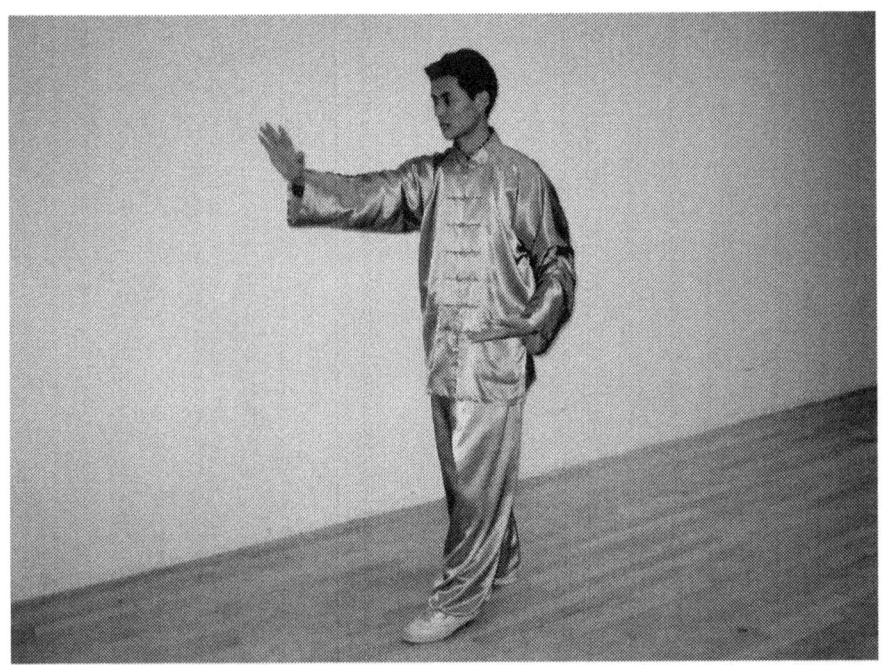

Pat the High horse

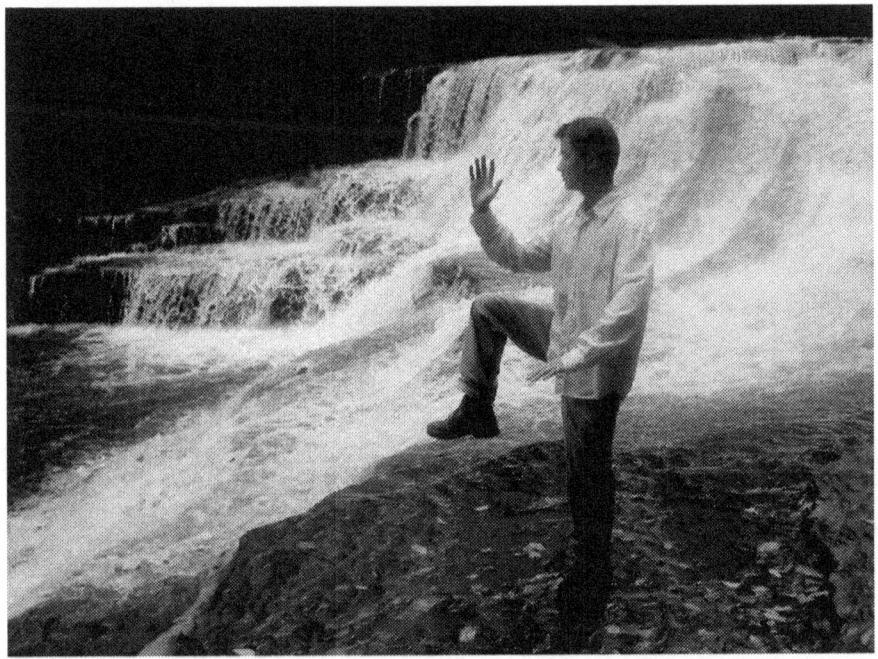

Golden Roster Stands With One Leg

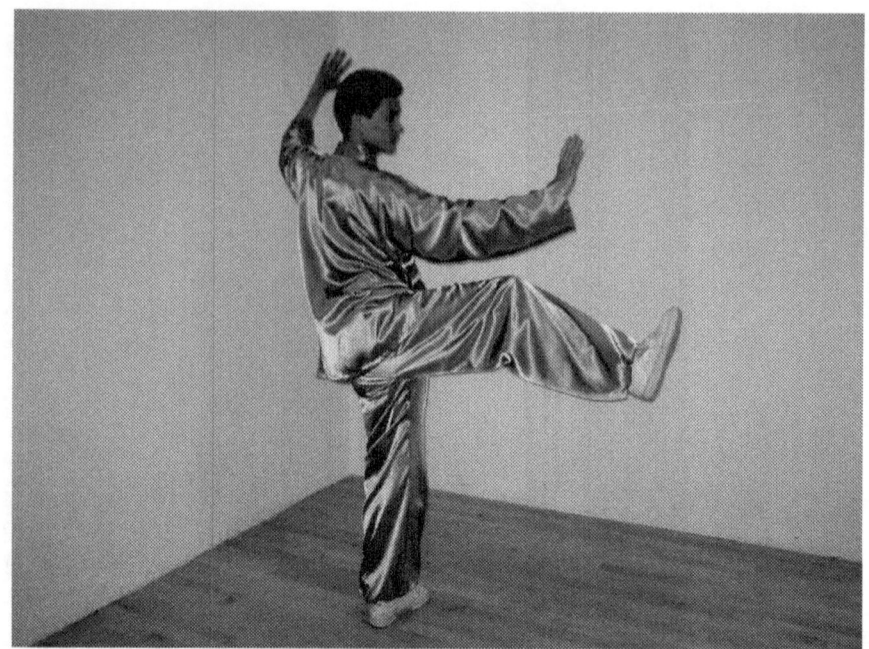

Right Heel Kick

6. Moving on Ice

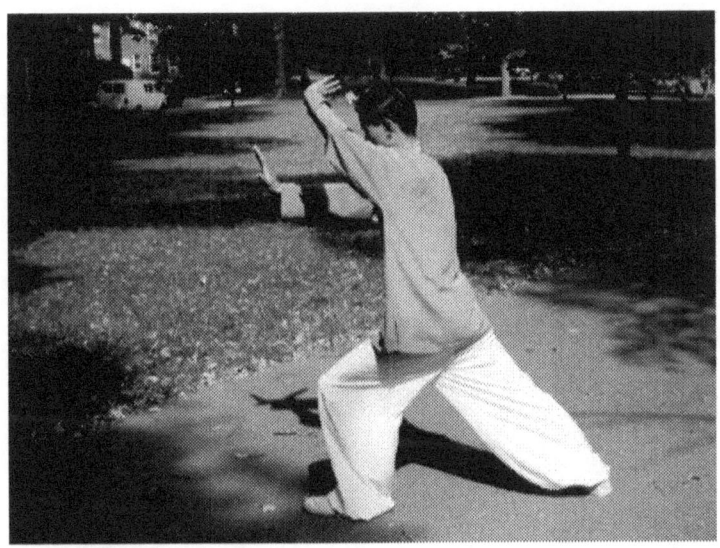

Huan putting his leg down carefully on jade lady works at the shuttles

"Wait for the chance to take a move (attack) like a cat's walk."

Zhang San Feng, the Creator of Tai Chi

"Moving on ice" or ice theory is another valuable principle about how to apply Tai Chi footsteps. Differing from the topic of the last chapter, ice theory concentrates more on weight control rather than accuracy. There are two images about ice that are used to aid Tai Chi movement. The first is the slipperiness of ice. The other is the care needed to keep from cracking thin ice.

Ice Theory involves training yourself to grab the ground with your feet and a little bit about foot positions. Since the root is very important to Tai Chi, weight control while stepping is extremely important for Tai Chi. To apply footsteps very well, you have to know about ice theory.

Walking on ice teaches you to distribute your weight evenly. It teaches you how to step onto the foot.

You have to step carefully as if you were stepping on thin ice. Also, if you are stepping on thin ice, this means that you have to position your foot slowly and carefully; otherwise, you will break the thin ice. You need to perform a good weight transition from one foot to the other.

You don't release your weight like external martial artists do where you put your weight suddenly and strongly on the ground. Put your weight on ice evenly so you won't break it.

Imagine walking on ice with an uncertainty of its thickness. As you place a foot for the next step, care should be taken by testing the ice to see if it can hold up your weight. The rear foot needs to keep the weight of the body while the front foot tests the ice. If the ice begins to give under the lead foot, the foot can be retracted easily because the body weight is still on the rear foot.

As the front touches and tests the ice, care is needed on how the weight is spread across the foot. If just the heel came down, it would exert much more pressure on the ice then if the whole foot were used. The more spread out the weight is, the more ice supports the body and the less likely that the ice will break.

The heel, the outer edge, and the balls of the feet should evenly press against the ground. The weight should even spread evenly across the balls of the feet from behind the big toe to behind the little toe. As you shift your weight to the front, the pressure needs to continue to build up evenly. The back foot should not release its hold of the body weight until the last moment.

Zhang San Feng's Tai Chi bible mentions walking like a cat. This means that you need to control your weight very well and not make any sounds while you make a move.

A common mistake is to step too quickly without a gradual transfer of weight. This can be observed if you make a big sound when you step down.

Since the ice is very slippery, you need to be very careful and slow down your step so you won't slide and fall down. In order to do that, you need to step carefully and grab the icy ground with your feet.

Some very good exercises to do in order to develop weight control is the transition from raise hands to white crane spreads its wings, fair lady works at shuttles, needle at the bottom of sea, step back to repulse the monkey. Pay close attention during these movements to how the weight comes down to the step foot and then to how the weight shifts to that foot.

In conclusion, this chapter teaches you to move the weight to the feet.

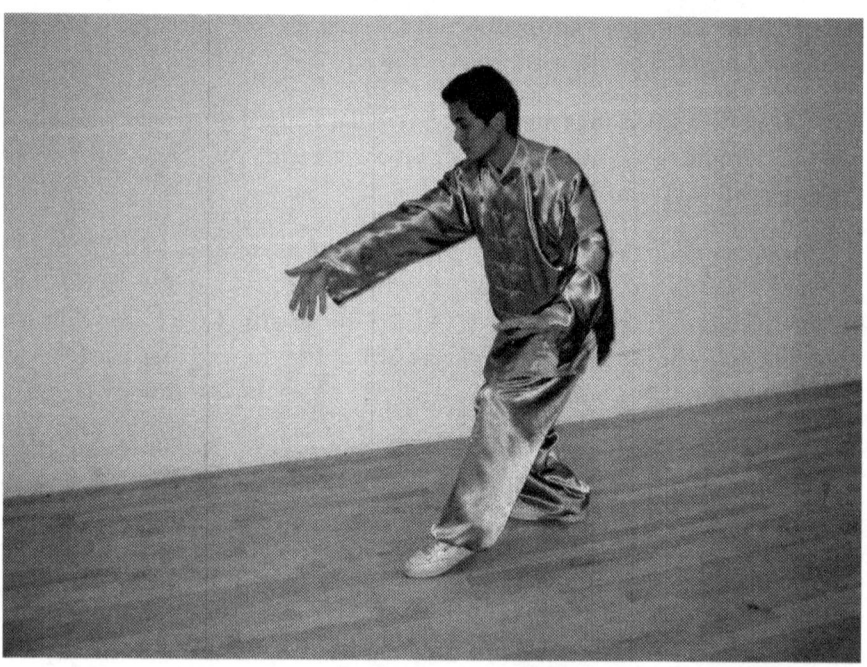

Needle at the Bottom of the Sea

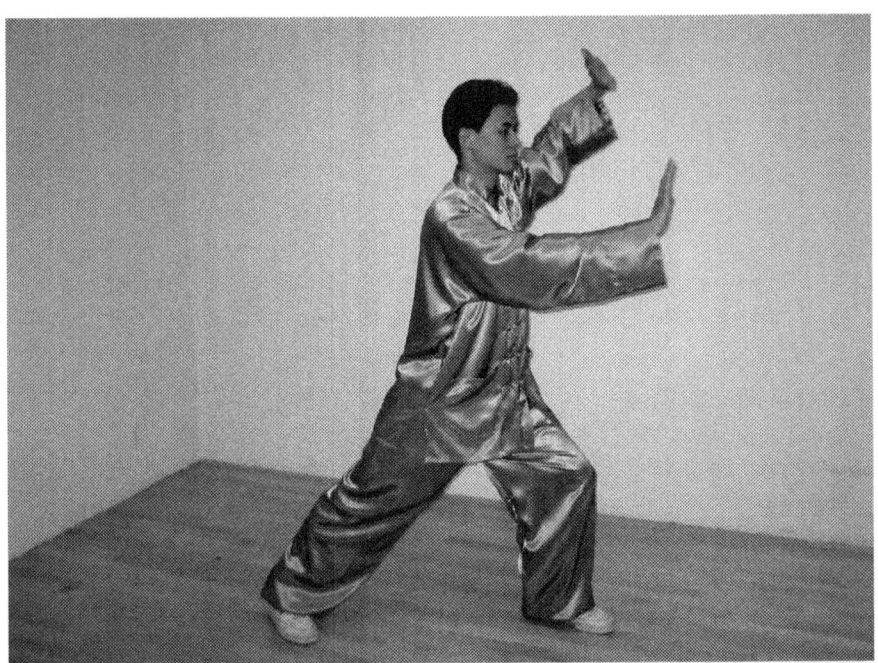

Jade Lady Works at the Shuttles

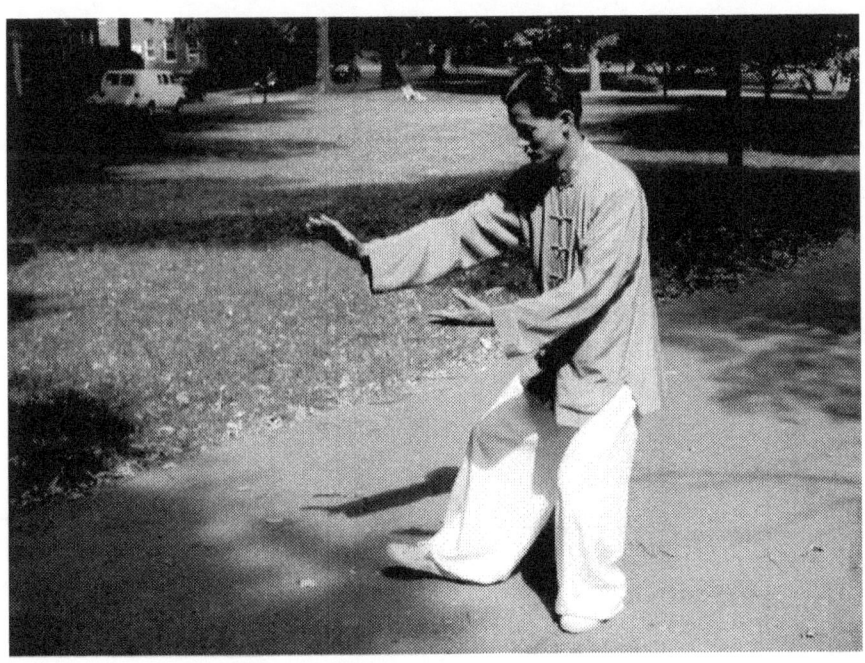

Repulse the Monkey

7. Raising the Feet from Mud

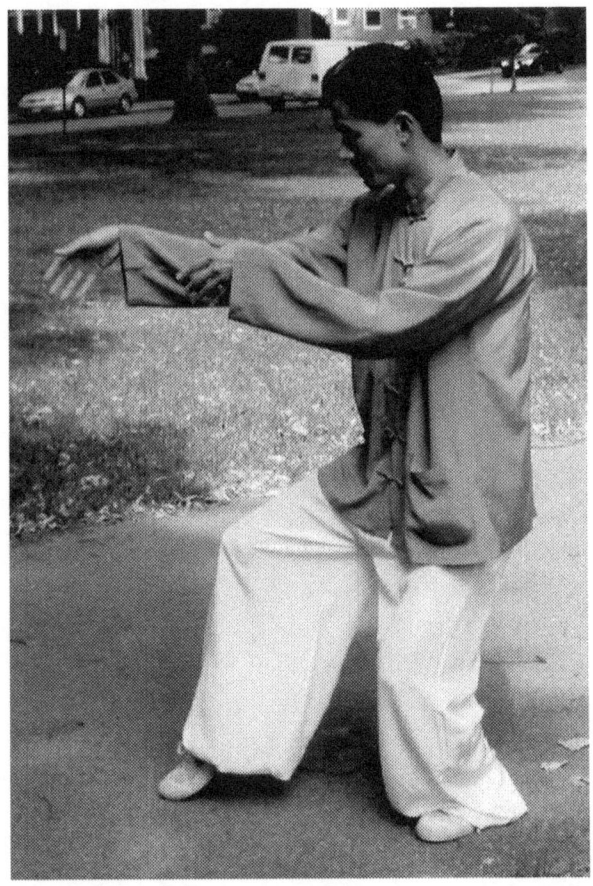

Huan Zhang apply mud theory while doing lifting hands.

> "Walking like moving in the mud."
>
> Unknown Martial Artist

Many external martial arts sets have this special step named "step in mud stance." It's usually a low stance that shows you the feeling of being stuck in the mud. As I practice Tai Chi, I discovered that the mud stance was very useful in Tai Chi as well.

The mud theory applies sticking technique to your feet. It lets you have the ability to feel the control of your feet. It teaches you that you should not slide your feet while you are moving. Your feet should be taken out of the mud and put into the mud. It makes you feel connected with the ground. Your feet are taken from the ground but are also connected to the ground.

> "Five toes grab the ground."
>
> Zhang San Feng

When you try to raise your foot, you have to feel like you are taking your legs from mud. You move the weight little by little from the ground. You need to feel the stickiness of the ground. Zhang San Feng said that the toes of the feet have to grab the ground. Only if they grab the ground will you have a good weight center and your body will have good balance and connection with the ground.

For example, Zhang used cat walking to show Tai Chi walks. The walk has to be light, quiet, but also have this stickiness to ground. It teaches you not to move your weight quickly from the ground--it has this grabbing power. You have to feel like taking it out of the mud, slowly, and heavily. My father always told me, when you practice, while you take your foot up, you should feel like you are raising a thousand pounds. It's so heavy and hard to even move your leg. So when you bring it up, you don't bring up right away. You try to release it from the ground gradually, feeling the weight release in ever decreasing pressure until the foot is free. Such exercise requires good strength, patience, and good imagination.

Let us now talk about how to put your feet and legs into the mud. Slowness is always the key. You shouldn't put your feet into the mud too quickly; that would allow you to transfer your weight too fast. Imagine if you put your foot very heavily and quickly into mud. It would squeeze and splash the mud. The mud would fly all over your face. You don't want this to happen, so you carefully and slowly put the leg/weight little by little onto the ground. Thus, most times you should first use the heel of your feet to first touch the ground, and then put the weight down by slowly increasing percentage until it reaches the full 100%.

A good exercise is lifting hands; remember that while you are doing lifting hands you have to lift your legs as well. Golden cook stand with one leg is another great exercise for practicing the mud technique. Simple but complicated moves like brush knee always can be used as practice footstep theory like mud theory. Pay attention to how the how the foot comes off the ground. With brush knee, pay attention to how the foot lower to the ground.

Note that "Walking on the Edge" theory talked about the care needed in placing the foot. The "Ice" theory talks about how to bring the weight to the foot. The "Mud" theory talks of how to lift the foot and how to bring it down.

8. Becoming Water and Waves

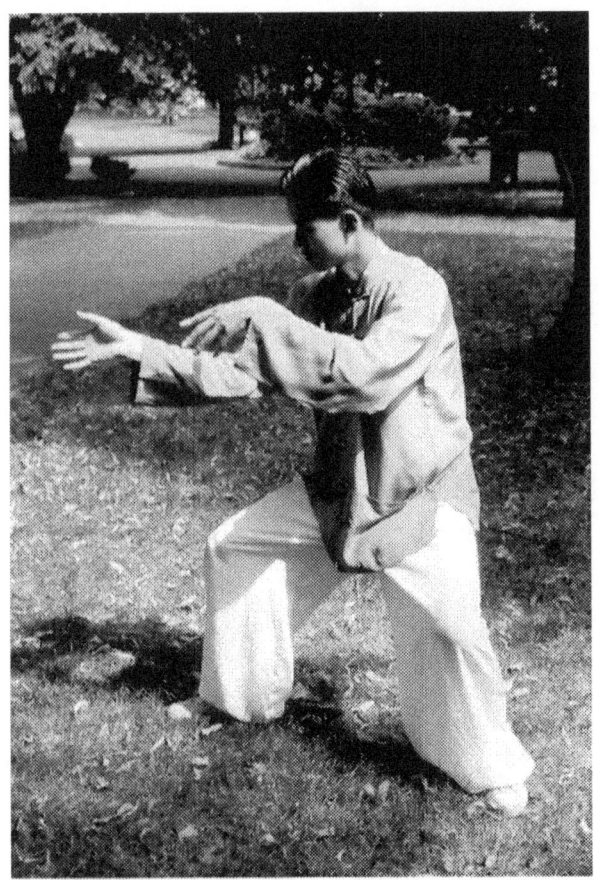

Huan applies water theory while perform Lu.

"Quiet like Mountains, moving like rivers."

Wang Zhong Yu, Originator of Tai Chi

Perform Your Tai Chi in Water

The water theory teaches you to feel resistance while you move your body. It develops a natural response to both the internal and external forces that are around us. It develops an understanding of how to gather the energy throughout our body and focus them into a single powerful force.

The water theory teaches you that you should feel like you are practicing in water. You need to do the movements slowly, with a feeling of resistance. The Qi or water will be all over you. You need to feel light and relaxed but not like you are floating up above the water. You need to develop a sensitivity that is acute enough to even sense the air that surrounds you. You need to be able to sense the slightest internal tightness that resists the movements of our bones.

Also, imagining that you are practicing in water teaches you not to move in a straight line but to use a curved direction. Because of the water resistance, you have to move on a curve; otherwise, you will experience large resistance. In an actual application, if you move in a straight line it is very easy for your opponent to predict your move whereas a curved movement is more mysterious to him.

The Qi that flows out of the practice of water theory can impact your opponent strongly. Also, it will be easy for you to absorb his energy since his Qi will follow your Qi because your Qi is stronger. A larger amount of water overtakes the smaller one.

Steps in water need to be slow and accurate. Every step you take, you move your legs and feet with the moving of Qi. So you will have strong Qi in your root/feet.

A few good exercises in which to practice the water theory is the "Step up to parry and punch", "Turn to side and punch", "cross hands" and "raise hands". As you do these movements, imagine the feeling of the resistance of the air as if it was water. Imagine the buoyancies that would affect your body if you were in water.

A couple of mistakes are to raise your arms too fast or to move in a straight line. Pay special attention that you avoid each of these pitfalls.

It is a good example to consider the power of Tai Chi as Waves. Waves smash stones. This is an example that compares internal martial arts to external martial arts. The internal martial arts such as Tai Chi are like waves while the external martial arts are more like stones.

The legend of "Huge Wave"

I read a Buddhism holy work one time. There is a very interesting story I like to use to describe the Tai Chi power - Wave. There is a famous wrestler of that time. His nickname is huge wave. How did he get this nickname?

It was because something happened to him that really bothered him. He had great skills and outstanding knowledge of wrestling, but, in real fighting, he always lost. Sometimes he couldn't even beat his student.

He was very bothered, so he went to a very high mountain to this mysterious monk. The monk told him a way to get back his confidence. When you move your body, you need to imagine yourself as a big wave with infinite power that can smash the whole world. All other opponents compared to you are nothing.

After he went back to his normal life, he won almost every battle. The wave theory really works. So he got a nickname "Huge Wave."

This story tells you how waves can be so powerful if you imagine it when you practice. Sometimes, people mistakenly don't concentrate when they imagine it. They need to concentrate on it; so all the water came together to form the huge (infinite) wave and smashes everything.

The water theory also really trains your patience, tolerance, and the mind control of your foot movements. It gives great ideas of how to raise, move, and put down your feet. The correct footsteps determine the whole movement of Tai Chi. Without the correct steps, your Tai Chi will become handicapped. With the theory of Water you will do better on Tai Chi footwork.

On the other hand, the wave theory builds your concentration, your strength, and your confidence. With such a big influence of the huge wave, you can smash everything on earth with it; thus you build a very strong Qi that strengthens your body and mind.

9. Using Good Imagination

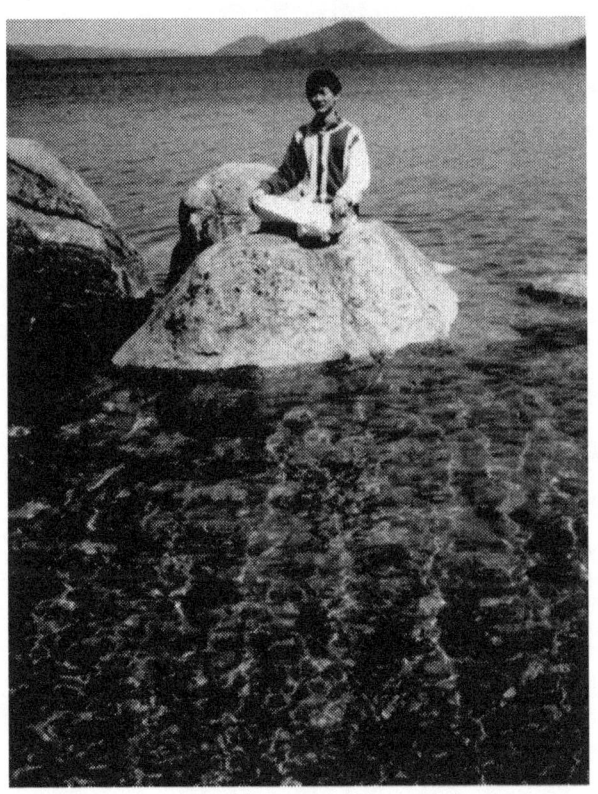

Huan Zhang uses imagination to meditate.

"Tai Chi is a way to recapture the art of soft breathing and calmness that we associate with the young. It's all about your state of mind as well as the state of your body."

Lu Ping Zhang[7]

The Father and Son Talk on Imagination

I remember how my father and I spent a lot of late nights discussing some Tai Chi theories. It was hard to get his compliments since he was kind of strict and tried to be perfect in all the theories. However, he developed my imagination for Martial Arts and Tai Chi. He told me that if I used my imagination and creativity with a combination of his scientific proofs and experience, we would find a new way to explain Martial Arts. I should not do the traditional way of just following the teacher to learn it and of just trying to memorize it.

He told me that, "Some day, when I am not doing mathematics research any more, I want to put my time into organizing all the martial arts theories that I know. And use my own knowledge to rework all the martial arts sets to make them more understandable by using many examples such as imagination."

"I have many new ideas about Tai Chi which come to mind every day. I just don't have enough time to write them down." He said.

Since when my father was very young in college, he was able to study with a number of grandmasters. After each training session, he would come up with more uses beyond those that the grandmaster taught him. From every application he learned, he was able to use his imagination to make more and better applications. He always encouraged his students to use their minds to think to make better movements themselves but use the scientific way to verify them.

How Imaginations Help You on Tai chi

As you have read so far in this book, you have seen that many examples that I use are from my imagination. They are intended to aid you in your own imagination in ways that will help you do Tai Chi better.

Let us consider some examples of using imagination to improve ones Tai Chi. When you move your hands you can imagine that you are moving your hands along a big ball. This vision will make your movements more smooth and round.

Let us explore the vision of taking a shower in the morning. You can imagine how the water runs over your body. You can imagine how the spray gets into your skin and opens the pores in your skin. Just as actually being in the shower will relax you, the active imagination of that event can relax you. Maybe the similar image of standing under a waterfall works better for you. While you do your Tai Chi, you might imagine the waterfall is running over your head, down your shoulders, your chest, and your whole body. You might be drawn enough into the image to actually feel the weight of the water splash on you. The imagination might spark the feeling as if water was actually flowing down varying paths on your body. These images will help you to relax more. By developing further images in your own mind, you could find personal vision that will help you even more.

On the other hand, some bad images might be harmful to your Tai Chi. Consider when someone first learns how to do push hands. The student might imagine in their form that they are pushing hands with someone else. However, many people early concepts on push hand imagine conflict. This concept can only cause the movements both in their forms and in the push hands to become stiff and hard, not soft and fluid.

Another example of poor imagination is in losing sight of the actually movement. When you imagine moving like a cat, do not get lost in details of one cat's that doesn't belong in the movement. Just because you have seen a cat, arch its back in a certain way or bush against a wall, you should not imitate this behavior in doing your Tai Chi. You don't want to imagine too much. You might forget what the real movement is. You might forget that you are doing Tai Chi and concentrate too much on looking and acting like a cat. These bad images can interrupt the concentration on the movement and interfere with relaxation.

You should always use your imagination to expand your understanding of Tai Chi, but always keep sight of the principles of Tai Chi.

10. Blind Men Touch the Elephant

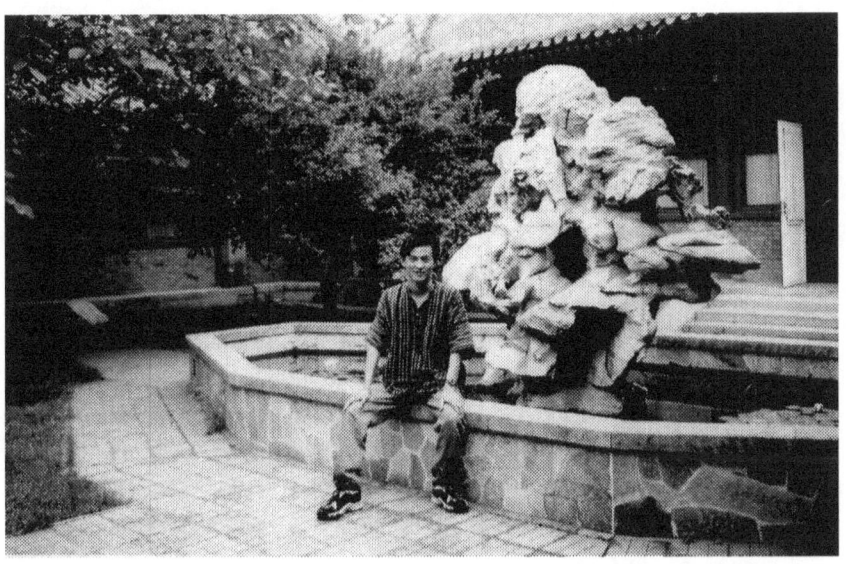

The shape of this stone looks different in each direction, so as Tai Chi.

Where is the Tai Chi Elephant?

> "Dao is the whole universe, like all the streams combine to be the ocean"
>
> Lao Tzu

Tai Chi has its own universe. It's contains its streams, and each stream is different. Without these different stream/ movements, the Tai Chi can't be Tai Chi.

There is an ancient Chinese story about four blind men describing an elephant. Four blind men came upon an elephant. The first blind man touched the leg, so he says that it is a big pole. The second man touched the tail, so he says that it is a snake. The third man touched the body, so he says that it is a wall. And the last man touched the ear and he thinks that it is a fan.

Since they only touch a part of the elephant, they still don't know what an elephant looks like. Tai Chi is like a huge elephant, some time it's easy to show a piece in detail but it is hard to give the whole view.

The Hundreds of Applications of One Movement

In some Tai Chi martial arts training, the movements in the forms have a very specific application. A specific response to a specific attacked is given as the intention of each movement. I have seen explanations showing how a long series of moves will defeat a particular attack. Each part of the form guides the opponent to a more detrimental position until the series end with his total defeat. I have seen training where these long series are practice repeatedly to develop an automatic response to a given attack. The partner will constantly make changes in the way he makes his attack in order to help the partner sharpen the effectiveness of his movements.

In an actual fight, it is hard to believe that a long sequence of movement could be maintained. There are just too many potential changes in a fighter's response to expect it to go to completion. In boxing matches, most fighters are looking for places in the opponent's pattern to take advantage of the routine.

To the other extreme, some Tai Chi instructors never show applications. They may not have been taught the applications, may not understand them, or may believe that learning the underlying principles are all that is needed.

Lu Ping loved to show a large number of applications for each movement of the form. He would say that he could show hundreds of applications for the smallest piece of a movement.

I can remember him showing an application where he captured a punch and threw the attacker to the side by redirecting the punch energy. The person was sure that he could make his punch in some way to defeat this application. The numerous attempts with different punches were counter in ways that threw the attacker in different directions. The person began to complain that Lu Ping wasn't using the same application against each of these attacks. Lu Ping explained that the punches were simply catching different parts of the same application.

This incident shows the various aspect of a single application. You should also consider the numerous reasons which people are drawn to Tai Chi. It is referred to as "Meditation in Motion", "Fluid Yoga", "The Supreme Ultimate Fighting Art", "Exercise for the Elderly", and various different descriptors. It is noted for reducing falls in the Elderly, throwing someone without touching, standing against the push of twenty opponents, promoting deep relaxation, overcoming illness, and improving health. The difficulties of seeing Tai Chi as a whole should be clear from this range of aspects.

When one of Lu Ping's students first began studying with him, he was very hesitant in doing martial arts applications. He had been only interested in the Energy aspects of Tai Chi and only wanted to learn the form to develop this skill. Lu Ping told him that if he wanted to learn the energy and health aspects of Tai Chi, he needed to even be more focus on the fighting skill. He said that it was also true that to develop the advance fighting skills of Tai Chi, one needs to focus on the Health and Energy aspects.

11. Finding the Right Transition

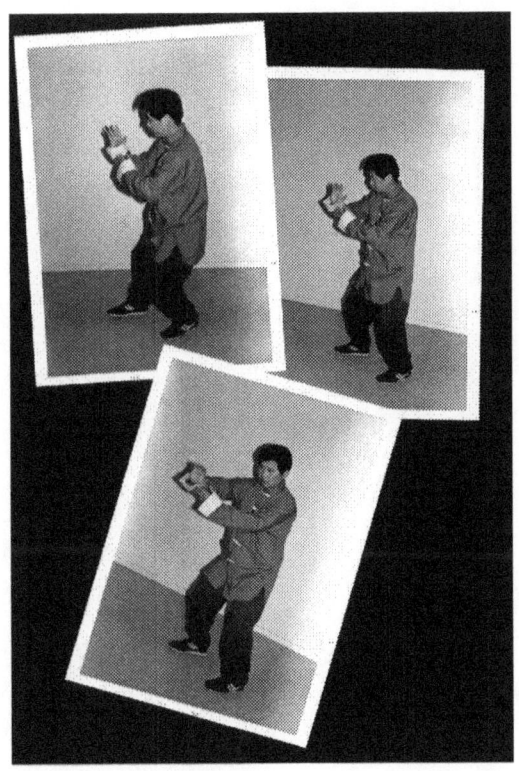

Master Lu Ping Zhang doing transition from Lifting Hands to Single Whip.

> "Tai Chi is like a long river; it brings waves and never stops."
>
> Wang Zhong Yu

Tai Chi, The Long River

"There are many talented people who can learn martial arts very fast, some can even learn by reading a martial arts book. No one can really learn the Yang Style Tai Chi from the book, because there is no picture of Yang Cheng Fu doing the transition movements. You need to learn the transition movements as close to original as possible." My father once told me this. The Transitions are so important and they are extremely hard to get. As Wang Zhong Yu said, "Tai Chi is like a long river; it brings waves and never stops."

Tai Chi is a martial arts set with continuous movements. In order to maintain continuous movements, we have to have good transitions. The many little complicated transitions such as from "lifting hands" to "White Crane Span its Wings" or the many easier transitions such as from "Getting the Needle from the Sea Bottom" to "Fan Through Back" are all important to the whole performance of Tai Chi. I have seen many people learn from books or low level martial arts schools; they have very bad transitions or almost no transitions at all. How can Tai Chi be Tai Chi if there are no transitions? Good transitions include feet moving, balance, and smoothness, the concentration of the eyes, and the understanding of the gesture.

The Smooth and Easy Transitions

To form smooth and easy transitions, first you need to know how to move your weight, as we mentioned above in the chapters in which we discussed the "Ice, Water, and Mud" theories. You basically know how to move the legs. The upper body and hands should be coordinated and move with legs as a whole unit. Do it slowly. Don't rush it and hurry on to the next movement. Each transition movement is as important as the standing gestures.

Balancing is very important in the transitions as well. Without good balancing the transition will look awkward. Balancing can make the gesture looks even and graceful.

My father used to tell me that I have to pay attention to each individual gesture. He wanted to make sure each of my gestures, which include the transitions, look good in the pictures. This emphasis doesn't mean that my Tai Chi had to look flashy; it meant it had to be balanced and smooth.

How to make your movement smooth: Just like your handwriting if the edge is rounded up, it looks smooth and nice. Making your movements in circles instead of straight lines can smooth your Tai Chi. That is why an internal martial arts set looks smoother than the external martial arts set. External martial arts set such as Karate teaches you how to punch straight and kick in a line, which is not smooth but sudden. To make it smooth, you need to curve it instead of forming a straight line.

Of course, the understanding of the gesture determines the right transition for each movement. Without really understanding the meaning of each movement, the transition you do will be meaningless since you have no idea how the transition goes and you are just doing the routine.

It can aid to learn numerous new positions between the main postures that are taught. They can serve as guidepost of how the transitions should be done, but the true transitions require an understanding of the essence of each posture that it connects.

12. Understanding Bows, Bows and More Bows

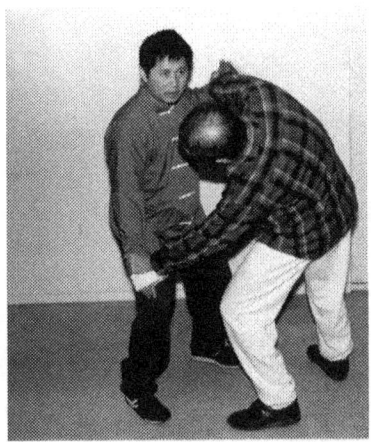

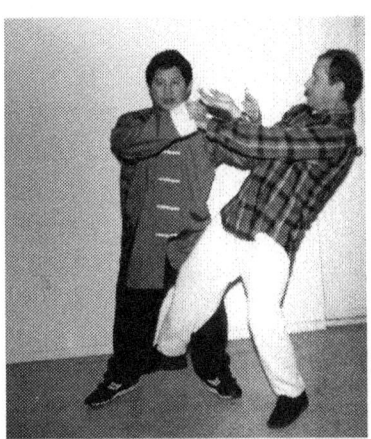

Master Lu Ping Zhang uses bow technique in push hands with
Tom Kimmerle.

"There can be many more than five bows, and they are used to focus the direction of force."

Lu Ping Zhang[8]

The Bow of Tai Chi

Unlike external kung fu that tries to straighten up your arms, legs, and whole body during the movements, Tai Chi is not straight and squared. Tai Chi is bent, curved and round. If a perfect shape were to be chosen for Tai Chi, it has to be round. When a shaped stone lay on the beach, the ocean will wash it and wear it into its perfect shape, round. When it is round, it is strong and it can move. When the powerful ocean wave came, the round shape will be maintained and it will keep itself in whole by moving around to avoid the huge ocean wave power.

This perfect round shape is a combination of many arches which also we call bows. There are 5 major bows in the Tai Chi forms. The two arms, two legs, and your spine each forms one of these bow to strengthen your structure and maintain your Qi and power.

As my father mentioned above, there are more bows; for example, your hands can form bows as well, your fingers can form bows, and even your feet and your toes. Each of these big or smaller bows supports your body and gives a good frame for your Tai Chi gesture.

"(When it is) Bent and curved, then it will keep (itself) the whole. Bent and stretch, then it can extend"

Lao Tzu

How Bows Work

Why bows? Bows are important because they are part of the circle. The bow can maintain weight or power (See Draw 12-1). When your body is squared and flat, a force apply to your body will concentrate and gather and bring it to the center of you body, thus hurt you. When you have an arch or bow, the roundness will evenly spread the power to the whole arch to smooth the power to just the surface of the body. The bow keeps the force from penetrating thus protecting the body.

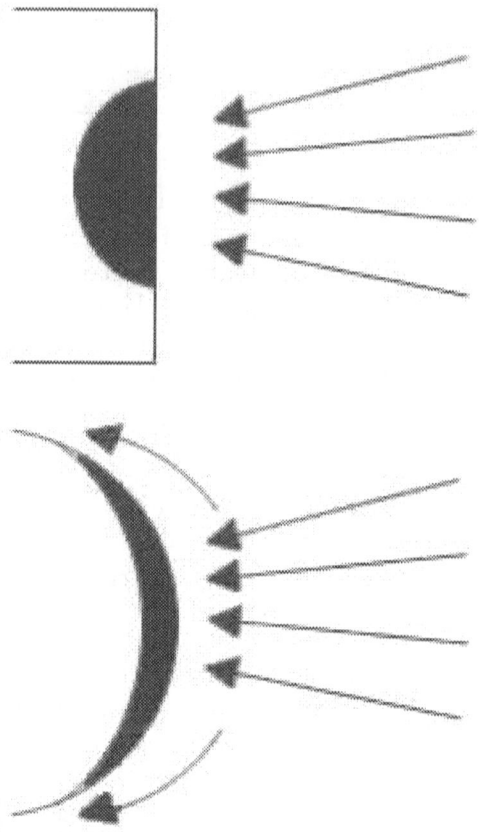

On, the other hand, the bow can store energy effectively as well. You can see how much power a bow can give when it shoots an arrow. It can go so much further then you could throw it. You do not even use electricity or fuel to shoot the arrow, but you can shoot something very far. That's the amazing thing about a bow.

My another Tai Chi teacher Xie also mentioned that if you have good stance and form good bows, then your stances are very stable and not easy to be pushed away in push hands. He first demonstrated it himself by forming strong bows and having students push at him. He then he adjusted a teenager student into such a stance, and asked a big person to push him but the small teenager couldn't be pushed away because the bow was so strong.

He had me form the stance called An (Push). He sat on my legs to show his students how strong my bow was. Even though I am a skinny person compared to Xie, my legs are strong enough to easily maintain his weight.

When I teach my students the theory of bows, I demonstrate it to them by teaching them how to form a good stance, form a nice strong bow stance, with bow shaped arm. When the students believe they have a good stance. I will test it by pushing each with big power to show them if their structure is able to resist power and stay strong.

The Farmer Who Pulls The Crops

I found that for some students when they try to do Tai Chi, they try to mimic the master to apply the "Turtle Back". Actually "Turtle Back" is the way of forming a bow on the spine. Trying to mimic and get the "Turtle Back" effects will not make your Tai Chi better, but it might misalign your spine. So mimicking "Turtle Back" is a very bad thing to do.

I have an example to show you: A long time ago in China there was a farmer. He planted a lot of crops. The crops grew very slowly every day. He wanted them to grow taller and faster, so he pulls each of them a little higher, and the second day he found all the crops dead.

So "Turtle Back" is the same thing. That's one of the bow things we don't want to get right away. How do advanced martial artists form a "Turtle Back"? It comes out automatically after years and years of practicing Tai Chi and other martial arts, so it will come. You just need to practice more.

To develop proper bows, it requires that proper attention be played to the shape. As you practice, you will start to notice a natural bounciness in your body.

13. Seeing the Long Hook within the Owl's Eyes

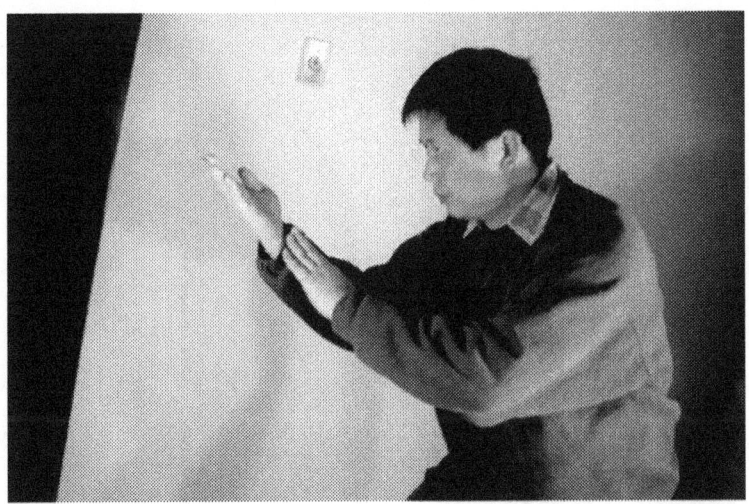

Master Lu Ping Zhang use eyes to apply concentration in Tai Chi.

"Your 'xing' is like an eagle that is going to catch the rabbit. Your 'shen' is like a cat that is going to get the mice."

Wong Chong Yu

Xing and Shen

Approximately four hundred years ago, Wong Chong Yu, the originator of Tai Chi, wrote the above quote in his Book of Tai Chi. "Xing" refers to your structure and how the movements appear from the outside. "Shen" refer to your concentration, eyesight, spirit, and how the movement is controlled from inside.

We often use the cat's eye as an example to apply in Tai Chi theory. The eyesight needs to perform like the eyes of a cat that is going to catch a mouse. It is strong, powerful, and focused. My grandmaster Cai also taught me to use eagle's eyes to apply in external martial arts sets such as Sho Lin or Karate. Eagle's eyes are also a good way to describe it since it looks further and can see more and smaller details of small animals far away on the ground.

Both cat and eagle's eyes can be very useful to Tai Chi practice. "What can be the best way to describe Tai Chi eyes?" I thought, "It has to be the combination of the two, cats and eagles' eyes." I think an owl's eyes at night are theoretically the combination of cat and eagle's eyes. So the eyes we use to apply in Tai Chi should be used as "owl's eyes at night."

Why are eyes so important to Tai Chi? I learned many other martial arts sets when I was a little boy before I got into Tai Chi. My father taught me Tan Tui, breaking the movements into much greater details than is usually given to this foundation form. He asked his teacher, the legendary Hua Mountain Style Grandmaster Cai Feng Xiang, to correct my gestures. Cai emphasized the use of the eyes. In order to develop power, the shen or the sight of eyes must be strong. To develop strong shen, all martial arts forms must train the eyes to lead the hands. Hook means the shen is strong and is able to take in/absorb and destroy other people's energy.

In Tai Chi, there are many movements that help train the eyes to lead your hands. Some good examples are "single whip", "wave hands like moving clouds", "left and right knee kick", and "punch downward". All these movements are also a part of developing one's skills as a martial artist.

To use Tai Chi as a martial art, you have to do more than lead your hands with your eyes. You need to also always concentrate on the opponent's movements. The combination of leading the hands with the eyes and of focusing on the opponent helps to focus the whole body in the martial art application.

Since the Tai Chi Form is practiced solo, you might wonder how you would focus on the opponent's movements. The solution is to recognize how each movement would be applied to a person and imagine that opponent clearly in front of you. The eyesight should be positioned on this invisible dummy. Each part of the Tai Chi form should be performed carefully with the eyes concentrated with an awareness of how this invisible dummy is being manipulated by these movements. It is amazing how, by using clear intent, this invisible opponent can deepen one's understanding of Tai Chi Principles.

Without concentration of the eyes, the movements of Tai Chi are handicapped. A lot of people when they try to relax, they close their eyes. This is totally wrong. Learning to relax does not mean that you should close your eyes and do "blind Tai Chi". If one of my students closed his eyes, I would remark, "I didn't plan to give you sleeping lessons. Use your eyes."

Eyes lead the 'Qi' and 'Yi', the power and mind concentration of your body. They control the body's energy. When a person has a lot of energy, the eyesight is strong and powerful. On the other hand, when a person has less energy, his eyes look tired. The eyes also lead the energy. By moving the eyesight, the energy moves. When the eyesight stops at a point, the energy stops at the same point. If the eyes become stagnant at a point, then the energy becomes blocked. Your eyes have locked up your energy.

Now we are going to explore another very interesting topic. How can you use your eyes to lock and control your opponent's energy?

> "The most advanced stage of martial arts is to defeat the enemy with your eyes without even fighting."
>
> Grandmaster Cai Feng Xiang

Defeat the Enemy with Your Eyes

An experienced opponent usually concentrates on your eyes trying to figure out what your next step will be because the eyes show one's intentions. Having strong and confident eyesight can really destroy the confidence of your opponents. Before fighting with you, they will already doubt if they are really good enough to match up against you. Eyesight should be like a flashlight that has come out at night. It can scare the opponent. On the other hand, half-closed or tired eyes will increase their confidence in defeating you. To strengthen your eyesight, you can perform in front of a mirror. Compete with your own eyesight in the mirror and see who has the stronger eyesight, you or your reflection.

An advanced way to perform Tai Chi is to expand the eyesight. When people did Push Hands with my father, they were always so amazed that even though he was so much shorter and smaller than the American guys, he could push them so far. They would wonder, "How could he possibly do that? What is his secret?"

One secret that I'm revealing to you is the use of the eyes. The eyes of Tai Chi are the vanguard of 'Yi.' To push away a person, you have to apply your Yi to him. To push him away further, you have to look at where the power needs to go. By using your eyes, you can double or triple the power applied whether it is your own power or his power reflected back at him.

To push far, you first need to have a good structure. For example, when using 'peng,' you need to have your peng shaped correctly. Next, you need to relax. Then you have to use your eyes and look to where the power will go. Finally, you can apply Yi and send the power to that point that you are looking at. If you look further, you will send him further.

There is a famous saying by a Chinese poet, "Bright sun falls down by the mountains, Yellow River runs into the ocean, if you want to see thousands of miles away, you need to go one more floor higher." To paraphrase this saying: to see with your own eyes the beautiful scenes in the distance, you must reach further.

A mistake you can make for using too much eyesight is to move your head too much; your head has to be centered and your chin has to be relaxed; also open your eyes don't mean to open them very wide and stare.

As a conclusion of this chapter, you need to bring concentration to your eyes while you perform Tai Chi. You need to follow your eyes with all your movements. You want to look beyond the movement of your hands in the direction you make your movements heading to, so the movement and concentration can be coordinated and become one. As we mentioned that Tai Chi is an exercise or martial arts set that requires the movement of the whole body and not the movements of a single part. Combining the eyesight movements to the whole body movements is a very important matter in Tai Chi training.

14. Knowing the "S" and the mirror of "S"

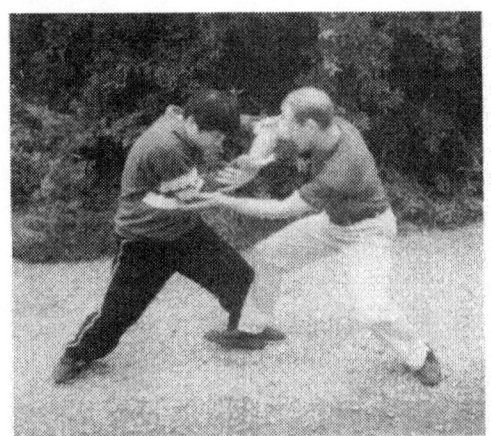

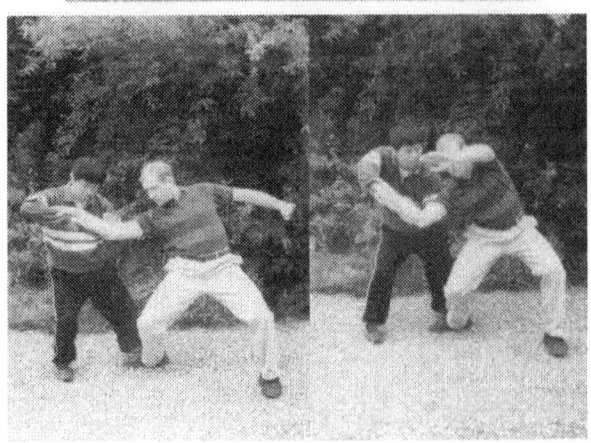

Master Lu Ping Zhang uses an "S" Curve with Tom Kimmerle.

"If you want to shrink it, you must open it. If you want make it weak, you need to strengthen it. If you want it to fall, you must raise it. If you want to take over, you must give all." Lao Tzu

The Ever-changing Curves of Tai Chi

Many people get confused when they hear the concept of the "S" line. Their perspective is just limited to a flat surface. They lock their concentration on the surface of the "S", the shape, and path. Truly understanding the "S" involves an understanding of the logical theory about the direction of force and its connection with the mind thinking and the human body responses. This is actually an advanced understanding of Dao.

A common martial arts principle that my father taught me is "First move right if you want move left." If you are already on the left, then you cannot move to the left. In Tai Chi, this principle applies easily to push hands (an exercise where two people try to feel each other's force and redirect their opponent's force). If you intend to move your opponent to the left, you should lead him to the right first. After he finds out that you are leading him right, he will counter the force by pushing back to the left. Now, his force is going to the left. It's your turn to help him move to the left direction as you planned at beginning. In order to do this task smoothly, you need to gather your movement into a curve.

The Two Strategies

We expands the above explanation into steps:

My Plan with Curve: Move him/her right and unbalance him.

My Step One: Move him/her left.

His/her step one: pull right (his left as he is facing you) to counter your force.

My step two: Follow his force to bring him to the right as my plan.

We all know that curves are better than straight lines, because they are unpredictable. These curves might still be predictable to intermediate-level and advanced level Tai Chi performers. However, the "S" line theory can be more unpredictable, because it contains two curves with opposite directions. Their force are still continues and they are still in balance when you bring them to

91

left. To make them lose balance to follow the direction you want. We need to change the plan.

My New Plan with "S": Move him/her left and unbalance him.

My Step One: Move him/her left.

His/her step one: Pull right to against your force.

My step two: Follow his force to bring him to right.

His/her step two: Pull left to against your force with his last strength.

My final step: Follow his force to bring him to left as my plan.

As you can see that the new plan is little more complicated. It's a movement of the "S" line. It moves left=> right =>left.

What is the advantage of "S" line? Instead of making a curve in the Tai Chi movement with your hands, you try to make it two curves to form the "S" line, to completely take away the other person's force and lead him in an unbalanced way. You can even take other people's force and translate back to him or to nothing.

You should beware of potential mistakes that can occur when you do the "S" line. If the first curve and second curve are so equal, it will allow the enemy to be aware of your attack and the response to the expected force that it will use. The "S" curve can be made even more difficult to follow by moving it out of the plane so that it ends up either higher or lower than the beginning movement.

I have found it useful to expand my father idea to consider the mirror of "S" which is similar to "S" line, but it runs to the opposite way. By freely moving along these curves with changing sizes and planes, you develop the ability to generate ever-changing curves. If you can combine both "S" and the mirror of "S" to your push hands routine, you can make so many different changes in push hands. These push hands technique will improve your ability in no time at all.

15. Forgetting Everything

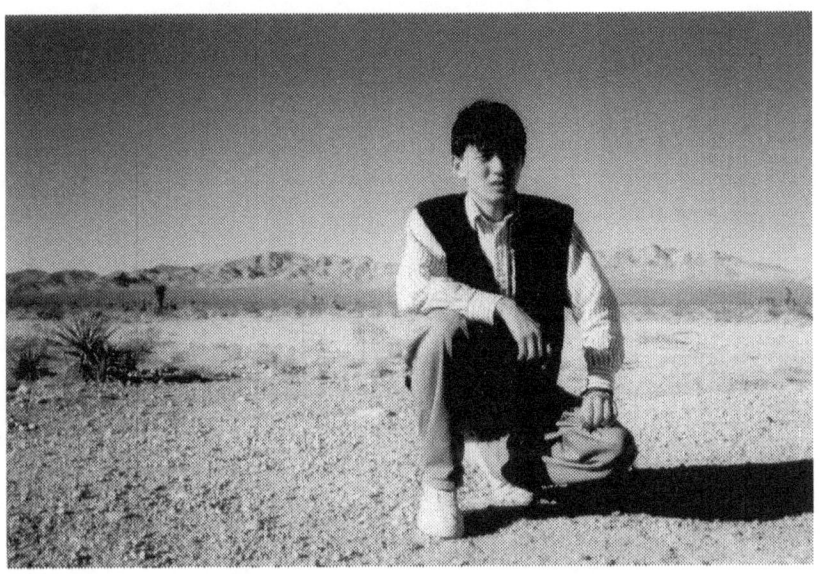

In a desert, there is nothing left but empty space.

> "When you succeed, try to think that it's not enough success, and then you will never stop succeeding. When you are filled with the Dao, empty it, then you can use the Dao forever"
>
> Lao Tzu

Free Yourself from Your Learning

If you already have your own idea, then new ideas won't come into you. If you really want to learn something new, you need to absorb it without prejudices and evaluate its truth. You must realize that what had work for someone else may not work for you and that even what had worked for you earlier, may no longer be correct.

I remember seeing Lu Ping teach three of his close students. He was working individually on the details of a movement. He showed each of them distinctly different details. One of the students couldn't quite get what he was being shown and started imitating the details that had been shown to another. When Lu Ping turned back to him, he admonished him that he was doing it wrong and again repeated the way he had earlier shown him.

Each of these students had their own difficulties in getting the essence of the movement. Lu Ping could see the different emphasis which each needed to progress and showed the correct details to that individual. The students would be wrong if they tried to do the other's details because it would move them away from the balance that they needed to gain the essence of the movement.

Lu Ping's Way

One of my father's early students in America told me about his frustrations when he first started studying with Lu Ping. He had studied Tai Chi for years and was teaching classes. Some of his students had seen Lu Ping and were especially impressed with his push hands. He took some public classes and saw that Lu Ping had great skill.

When he took his first private lesson, Lu Ping asked him to do his form. After he had barely gotten into the first movement, Lu Ping stopped him and said, "There are so many problems, I don't know where to begin". Lu Ping made a number of adjustments and then demonstrated how much more effective the movements were.

No matter how much you learn there is more to learn. In fact, you have to keep what you already know from interfering with your progression. I have had a couple of Lu Ping's students tell me how much they had to constantly change the way they were doing the form.

Lu Ping loved to get into arguments about Martial Arts. I remember Lu Ping telling me that none of the principles of Tai Chi were valid. For instance, the shoulders are not supposed to be behind the hip. He would then lean back and challenge people to push him. He would laugh when they failed to push him and yell, "See all principles are wrong".

Lu Ping was constantly looking to learn more. He was always looking to what other people knew even if he could see weakness in some aspects of their art. He was constantly testing these ideas with his students and testing his views. It is an approach that could help anyone expands his or her knowledge.

V. Epilogue and the 16th principle - Huan's Happy Tai Chi Theory

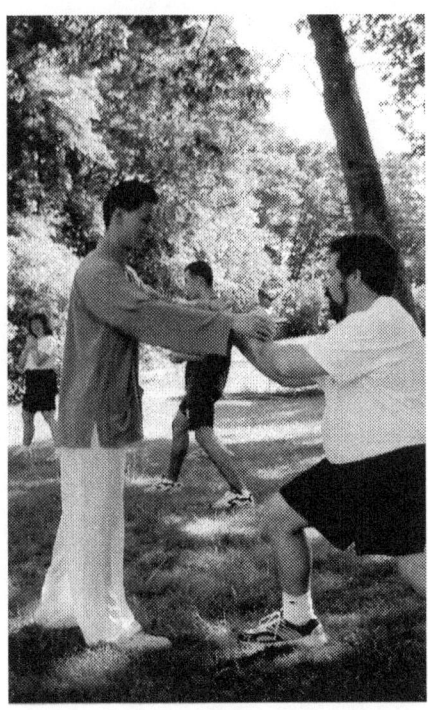

Huan Zhang correcting student's gesture

"If you are satisfied (with your Tai Chi), you are finished."

Lu Ping Zhang[9]

The thing I most often tell my students in Tai Chi class is to relax. To relax yourself, you need to start to relax from the head. Relaxing the muscle around the face is the first thing you need to do. After you have done that, your face will automatically form a smile. It's called the Tai Chi smile. After your smile has come out, you know you are happy when you do Tai Chi. You find your smile in your Tai Chi because you know that happy things happen to you when you smile.

Some people believe that Tai Chi is a hard thing to learn. And it is hard in some ways. They are not happy with their current level and feel that they should improve. My father used to say, "If you are satisfied (with your Tai Chi), you are finished." It means you can't improve your skill if you feel satisfied. A positive mood doesn't mean you feel satisfied with your Tai Chi. You need to have a positive mood to learn Tai Chi faster. You need to always feel good about yourself doing Tai Chi and believe that you are improving every day. And you are surely improving if you do it one more time, and you are getting to know the routine better.

I have told my students to think about Tai Chi as a happy and fun thing to do. It's a thing we can enjoy for our whole life because performing Tai Chi can make you smile and feel relaxed. It's such a pleasurable thing and it makes you feel good that you know your body will be healthier and you will improve your skills. Using my happy Tai Chi theory will make you perform Tai Chi with a positive attitude and make your Tai Chi learning process faster and more pleasant.

VI. One more thought • • •

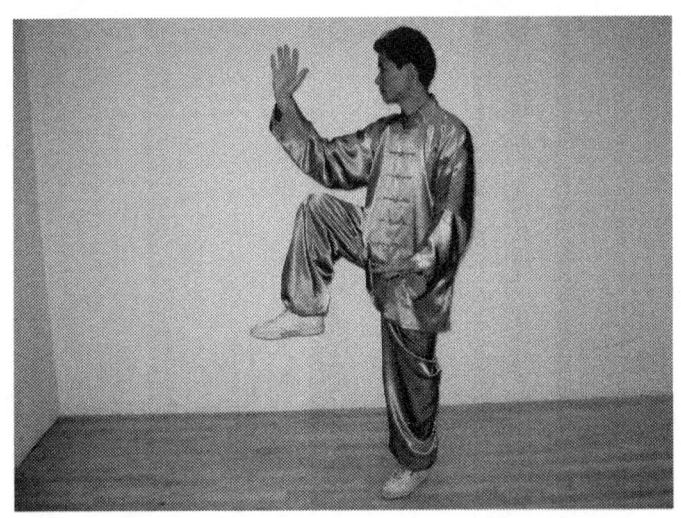

Here is an interesting and surprising way to improve your Tai Chi. Close your book and your eyes now. Open both the book and your eyes and look at the theory I mentioned on that page. Do the theory as the book says.

You are on your ladder climbing to the new stage of Tai Chi now.

VII. Honoring the Dead horse

When I was a child, my father told me this story. "An emperor wanted to have a good horse which could run for a thousand miles, but he didn't know where to get one. He spent a lot of money and bought a dead horse, which had run a thousand miles. People who owned such horses were very impressed by his sincerity and the honor he had bestowed on such a horse. They brought their horses to the emperor. So by buying a dead horse, he got many of these horses that he had wanted.

I am sure there are many people who have such horses, good ideas for this book; I welcome your sharing them with me. Your suggestions will be helpful to my future improvement of this book or future books. I am currently running back and forth between Boston and Amherst. My permanent address is 82 Stony Hill Road, Amherst, MA 01002. My e-mail address is huanzhang2000@yahoo.com. I welcome your e-mail or snail-mail. Thank you.

End Notes

1. Dan Miller, Founder of Pa Kua Chang Newsletter. *"Zhang Lu Ping Demonstrates a Straight Forward Approach to Pa Kua Chang"* Pa Kua Chang Newsletter, Sep/Oct 1991, Vol. 1 No. 6

2. Teri Lynn Breier, *"China's Lu Ping Zhang: Teaching While Learning"* Inside Kung Fu Magazine, May 1989, Vol. 16, No 5.

3. Marvin Smalheiser, Founder of Tai Chi Magazine, *"Skill, Not Celebrity, Is Important"* Tai Chi Magazine, April 1990, Vol. 14. No 2.

4. William Phillips, *"Zhang Lu Ping on correct Use of Spine"* Tai Chi magazine. December 1997, Vol. 21 No. 6

5. B. Jones. Tai Chi Magazine, April 1990, Vol. 14 No 2.

6. Hong Ying Min, "The Discussion of the Cabbage Root", Ming dynasty

7. Steve Pfarrer, *"Sense of order and harmony - Math professor finds connection as Tai Chi Expert"* Daily Hampshire Gazette, Friday, April 21, 1995

8. Marvin Smalheiser, Founder of Tai Chi Magazine, Tai Chi Magazine, vol.21, No.1, February 1997

9. Teri Lynn Breier. *"Where Have All the Masters Gone?"* Inside Kung Fu Magazine, May 1989, Vol. 16, No 5.

Other books Huan Zhang plans to publish:

9 Advanced Tai Chi Principles

Brief Introduction: This book teaches you how to use techniques such as adjust your spine, stick, circle, follow and lead, listening power, use your dan tian and learn how to empty yourself and absorb other people's power.

Hug a Pine Tree

Brief Introduction: This book teaches you a simple yet affective Qi Kong exercise to teach you to breathe and relax better with nature environment.

Develop Shadow Kicks with Tan Tui

Brief Introduction: A detailed step-by-step instruction manual to teach you these ancient fundamental Chinese martial arts set that almost every Chinese martial artist has learned.

Recommendation

I have been studying Tai Chi since 1967 and have met many masters and students. Lu-Ping Zhang and Cheng Man-Ch'ing are the greatest masters I have ever encountered. Lu-Ping Zhang had an encyclopedic knowledge of several styles of Tai Chi, and gave detailed and knowledgeable correction of those forms. In addition, he had a deep understanding of the underlying principles, and unique insights into each of the styles he taught. Huan Zhang, as his son, and inheritor of his wisdom, shares his father's understandings in this book.

William C. Phillips,

President and Founder of the Patience T'ai Chi Association, Brooklyn, New York.

About The Author

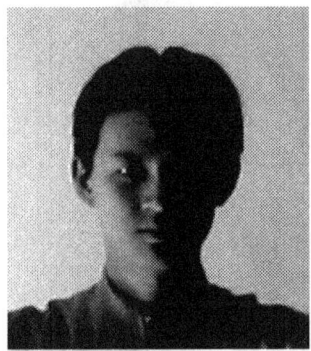

Huan Zhang

Huan Zhang is a teacher with an extraordinary background, who began studying Chinese martial arts in 1982. He has learned Tai Chi Chuan and other martial arts forms from his father, Master Lu Ping Zhang, Grandmaster Hong Xiang Cai, and Master Bin Can Xie. He has taught classes in both China and United States. He has assisted his teachers in the instruction of Tai Chi classes since 1989. Huan's articles have been featured in Tai Chi International Magazine.

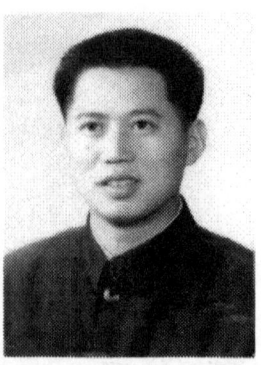

Lu Ping Zhang

He was a Math professor at both University of California in Irvine and University of Massachusetts in Amherst.

He has been a judge for many Tai Chi and Martial arts tournaments in both the United States and China. He was featured many times in a variety of magazines and newspapers: this includes being featured many times in Tai Chi magazine, including on the cover two times. Also featured in "Inside Kong Fu" magazine and "Tai Chi Combat" magazine in Austria Featured in TV shows such as "Full circle" for Tai Chi presentation.

He was a student of legendary Hua Mountain Style martial arts master Cai Feng Xiang, The famous "Little Tiger" Zhang Hai Seng. The "Great Power Wang (wang means king in Chinese)" Wang Zhi Ping, a legendary hero and warrior who survived the Boxer Rebellion in China corrected Lu Ping's Tan Tui. Dong Xiang Gen and Do Wen Cai, who are both students of Chen Zhao Kwei, also taught him. He also learned martial arts from many other famous and unknown masters.

www.ingramcontent.com/pod-product-compliance
Lightning Source LLC
Chambersburg PA
CBHW051438280526
45785CB00003B/1339